## BLACK HEALTH
## LIBRARY GUIDE

# STROKE

# BOOK YOUR PLACE ON OUR WEBSITE AND MAKE THE READING CONNECTION!

We've created a customized website just for our very special readers, where you can get the inside scoop on everything that's going on with Zebra, Pinnacle and Kensington books.

When you come online, you'll have the exciting opportunity to:

- View covers of upcoming books
- Read sample chapters
- Learn about our future publishing schedule (listed by publication month *and author*)
- Find out when your favorite authors will be visiting a city near you
- Search for and order backlist books from our online catalog
- Check out author bios and background information
- Send e-mail to your favorite authors
- Meet the Kensington staff online
- Join us in weekly chats with authors, readers and other guests
- Get writing guidelines
- AND MUCH MORE!

**Visit our website at**
**http://www.kensingtonbooks.com**

# BLACK HEALTH LIBRARY GUIDE

# STROKE

## Vital Health Information for African Americans

## LaFayette Singleton, M.D. with Kirk A. Johnson

Edited by Linda Villarosa
Nutritional Advisor, Maudene Nelson
Illustrated by Marcelo Oliver

KENSINGTON BOOKS
KENSINGTON PUBLISHING CORP.
http://www.kensingtonbooks.com

This book is not intended as a substitute for medical advice of physicians and should be used only in conjunction with the advice of your personal doctor. The reader should regularly consult a physician in matters relating to his or her health and particularly with respect to any symptoms that may require diagnosis or medical attention.

KENSINGTON BOOKS are published by

Kensington Publishing Corp.
850 Third Avenue
New York, NY 10022

First Kensington Printing: October, 1999
10 9 8 7 6 5 4 3 2 1

Printed in the United States of America

This book is dedicated to the memory of Gordon Banks, an African-American stroke patient and former athlete who died shortly after being interviewed.

Though partially paralyzed and confined to a wheelchair for years, he embraced life with courage and pride.

# Contents

# Foreword

Stroke may be one of the more misunderstood diseases of our time.

It's the third leading cause of death in the United States (behind heart disease and cancer) and the number one cause of disability in adults. Yet when a National Stroke Association survey asked Americans to name the leading causes of death, only 1 percent answered stroke.

Stroke is a condition that people equate with the beginning of the end. Once someone has a stroke, many assume the patient is beyond hope. But new rehabilitation therapies are helping more and more stroke survivors regain their former health. And exciting scientific discoveries are pointing to a day when doctors will be able to stop stroke dead in its tracks.

It's often considered an accident of fate or an act of divine intervention; the dictionary definition says the original meaning of the word "stroke" came from the phrase "the stroke of God's hand." Yet strokes are anything but random. As one researcher puts it, "Stroke is the end of a chain of events set in motion many years before." People can do a lot to make sure this chain of events never starts.

Stroke hits African-Americans harder than it affects almost any other people in the world. Compared to American whites, strokes in our community occur more often. And when they do, the damage is more severe. Rehabilitation is more challenging, and recovery is often slower.

We suffer more of the medical conditions that cause strokes, and we have less access to affordable, quality medical care.

On top of all that, we don't always have access to reliable information about stroke. We may hear that Uncle Lou's doctor warned him that he'd have a stroke if he didn't go back to taking his "pressure pills." But we may not understand how high blood pressure causes strokes, or why there's so much hypertension in the black community, or why so many African-Americans don't take their hypertension medicine.

We may know that Deaconness Jones down at the church had a "mini-stroke." But we may not realize what mini-strokes are, or why doctors say they're just as serious as a full-blown stroke.

We may have heard that African-Americans are prone to stroke. But we may not know why we are at special risk, or how to lessen our chances of having a stroke.

We may know that strokes run in our family. But we may not understand what makes one family more vulnerable than another, or we might be curious to find out exactly what our chances are of having a stroke ourselves.

We may be helping a loved one recover from a stroke, and we may wonder about the foreign-sounding medical terms that we hear in the hospital, or we may have questions about the procedures and medicines that the patient is receiving. Most of all, we may want to know what our loved one's prospects are for recovery and what to expect in the weeks and months ahead.

No book, including this one, can replace a medical professional. Only a doctor can diagnose and treat an illness, and only a doctor is qualified to pass judgment on an individual case. The information presented here cannot substitute for consulting with a physician or other health professional who is familiar with stroke and who knows a particular patient.

What this book does offer is information to help you make informed decisions about your health and the health of your loved ones. It's information designed to help you talk about stroke. If a loved one has suffered a stroke, this book will help you talk with doctors and will show how you can best help the patient. If you've had a stroke yourself, the book can help you make it through recovery.

The book is written specifically for African-Americans. Most books on stroke never mention black Americans, except in a passing remark on how blacks are at special risk of having a stroke. No one discusses the special challenges black people face in getting good medical care, or the unique ways that the African-American community pulls together to overcome adversity. No one interviews black doctors for their perspectives on what African-Americans should do to protect themselves from stroke, how blacks are affected when stroke hits a family member, and what black families should do to ensure that a stroke patient gets the best rehabilitation care. No one discusses preventing strokes from the perspective of African-Americans, whose views on preventive measures often differ from those of whites, and whose medical conditions may present special challenges to carrying out a sensible prevention program.

This book is intended to help fill that void. Inside you will find useful, informative material written for the lay reader. You don't have to know anything about stroke to benefit from this book. In fact, you don't need a medical or scientific background at all. The emphasis is on presenting up-to-date information in a nonthreatening, user-friendly format.

The book begins with "Straight Talk About Stroke." This opening chapter explains what a stroke is, how strokes happen, and which kinds of stroke are more prevalent in the African-American community.

Chapter 2 ("Black Folks at Risk") discusses over a dozen so-called risk factors that increase a person's chances of having a stroke and explains why black people are at special risk. At a glance, you can tell how important a risk factor is, how strong the evidence implicating it is, and whether or not a risk factor is preventable. With a little simple arithmetic, you can even calculate your (or a loved one's) chances of having a stroke.

Chapter 3 ("When Stroke Strikes") deals with stroke as a medical emergency. It explains the symptoms of someone who is having a stroke, and outlines the simple steps you can take to help him or her. This chapter also covers the procedures and tests that medical personnel use to help a stroke patient in the critical first hours. By explaining what constitutes good medical care and how the family can work with the medical team to benefit the patient, the chapter is geared to helping black stroke patients get the best possible care.

Chapter 4 ("Pushing Through Recovery") explains how the body and mind heal after a stroke. It will help you understand a patient's chances for recovery, and it explains the physical, mental, and emotional challenges faced by stroke patients and their families. The chapter highlights the special challenges that black stroke patients face during recovery, as well as the unique ways that the African-American family and community can assist.

Chapter 5 ("Prevention Is the Best Medicine") tells you how to prevent a stroke. It explains the medical options, including medication and surgery, for persons at high risk of a stroke. It also covers steps that virtually everyone can take to reduce their risk. One of the welcome benefits of stroke prevention is that when you reduce your chances of having a stroke, you also reduce your chances of having other diseases; this chapter explains how.

Chapter 6 ("New Hope, New Dreams") looks to the horizon to unveil recent research findings and new or experimental stroke treatments. It also discusses how many of these exciting new findings and treatments will benefit the black community.

At the end of the book, Appendix A explains some of the common myths about stroke and corrects certain misconceptions that are prevalent in the African-American community. Appendix B is a list of resources that can benefit stroke patients and their families. Many government and private nonprofit organizations are devoted to helping people prevent strokes and to supporting stroke patients and their families through recovery. Many offer free literature or advice for the asking, and some can put families in touch with support groups and others who can assist them through the difficult stages of rehabilitation. Appendix C helps you plan delicious, nutritious meals that will help prevent a stroke or help hasten recovery from one.

Finally, a handy glossary explains medical terms that may be unfamiliar to you.

We hope this book will play a role in black Americans' continuing quest for health and peace of mind.

LaFayette Singleton
Chicago, Illinois

Kirk A. Johnson
Champaign, Illinois
January 1999

# CHAPTER 1

# Straight Talk About Stroke

He set seventy-two records as a college athlete, and he was the first black man from his hometown to be drafted by a professional football team. But after years of dazzling performances on the athletic field, Gordon Banks faced his most strenuous physical challenge one August morning when he tried to get out of bed.

"I stood up, and my left leg was like a wet dishrag," the middle-aged father of four recalls. "I tried to stand again, but I fell across my wife's legs." Banks didn't understand what was happening to him, but his wife knew.

"Call the ambulance and tell them to come and get Daddy," she told the children. "He's having a stroke." Indeed, a massive stroke. In the blink of an eye, Gordon Banks had lost the use of nearly half his body.

Banks was confined to a wheelchair for the last 12 years of his life. But his spirits remained high, and he said he was making painstaking but steady rehabilitation progress, thanks to a lesson he learned as an athlete: Hard work eventually bears fruit. And he knew the value of prayer. "I'll tell you one thing, young man," he confided in an interviewer. "I know who made that grass green in your mother's backyard."

Of the thousands of black stroke patients across the country, Banks said he was one of the lucky ones. At least he could tell his story.

## WHAT IS A STROKE?

A stroke is an interruption of the flow of blood to the brain.

As everyone knows, the brain is our body's command center. It tells our heart to beat—and how quickly. It instructs our lungs to breathe—and how deeply. We cough or sneeze or yawn when we need to because our brains control these reflexes. The sense of balance a dancer needs to arch on tiptoe, the precise muscle-flexing that enables us to sit in a chair without toppling over—all of this comes from the brain. When we reach for an orange, our brain orchestrates a dialogue between the nerves and muscles in our eyes, arms, and fingertips. And when we take a bite, it's the brain that registers the cold and sweet and tartness from our mouths, coordinates chewing and swallowing, and starts the flow of saliva and stomach juices that begin digestion.

Although much of the brain's magnificence comes from its ability to direct the actions of dozens of muscles, nerves, and organs simultaneously, the brain is more than a master of ceremonies. It is also a vast repository of emotions, cravings, sensations, and intellect. The memory of our first kiss, the smell of fresh paint, the scratchy feel of wool are all embedded here. The brain is the organ of learning, whether the task at hand is riding a bike or reading a book. Through chemical messengers called hormones, the brain signals our urges for food and sexual expression. Each element of our personalities—generosity, temper, aggression, willpower—is stored in the brain.

The brain is hard at work every moment we are alive, from sometime before birth until the instant we die. Even when we're fast asleep, the brain continues to monitor all sounds, smells, and touches as if we were wide awake.

The human brain is clearly the most complex object in the world. It is infinitely more sophisticated than the most advanced computer, and yet the brain is much like a computer in one important way: the need for fuel. Without electricity, a computer would be nothing more than a lifeless box of circuits. The brain needs fuel, too, and it comes from the blood.

To understand how, it helps to appreciate a little anatomy. The human brain is made up of microscopic branching nerve cells called neurons (Figure 1) that are organized into units that perform specific functions. For example, our speech center is made up of millions of interconnected neurons that, like a library, store what we know about language. Neurons from our speech center are connected in turn to other neurons that form our memory, and to still others that control our lips, tongue, and voice box. When all of these functional units work in concert, we have the gift of speech.

Your brain contains a staggering number of neurons—perhaps one hundred billion in all. Scientists do not understand how this wrinkled gray mass of nerve tissue is somehow capable of such wondrously diverse tasks as, say, designing a house and appreciating the

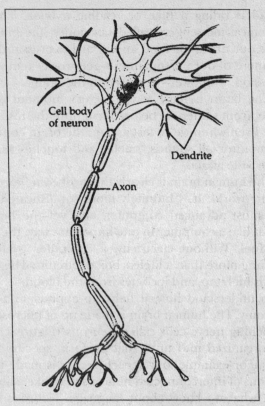

Figure 1. A nerve cell

subtle pinks of a rose petal. But they do know that the brain's nonstop activities demand an extraordinary amount of fuel in the form of oxygen, sugar (glucose), and certain other nutrients, all of which are transported through the blood. The adult brain weighs just three pounds—about 2 percent of your body weight. Yet the brain receives 14 percent of the blood flow and consumes a full 23 percent of the body's oxygen.

The delivery system for the brain's blood supply is understandably extensive. Each heartbeat sends blood streaming to the brain through the aorta, the body's main artery, and on to large arteries on both sides of the neck. These branch into smaller and smaller vessels, forming an elegant network of twisting, curving passageways (Figure 2).

By the time the blood vessels reach the innermost parts of the brain, they have become capillaries. These tiny channels are so narrow that four hundred of them placed side to side could fit on the period at the end of this sentence. Indeed, microscopic red blood cells often must squeeze through capillaries one at a time. It is in the capillaries that a crucial exchange of goods takes place. Oxygen and other nutrients from the blood travel through the wall of the capillaries and get delivered to individual brain cells. Meanwhile, waste products such as carbon dioxide and ammonia travel in reverse direction from brain cells to the capillaries, where they enter the bloodstream. The spent blood, including the newly acquired waste products, flows from the capillaries through increasingly larger veins in and around the brain and down through the neck. Eventually, the waste is disposed of through the lungs and the kidneys. Then the blood picks up more oxygen and nutrients and begins the cycle once again.

That's how the brain gets the energy it needs to direct the countless activities that make life possible and give it meaning. If that precious blood supply is disturbed, the results can be disastrous. The brain has such a relentless need for nutrients that if the flow of blood is interrupted by an obstruction or a leak, the brain tissue being fed by the blood vessel can start to die within minutes. When that happens, whatever

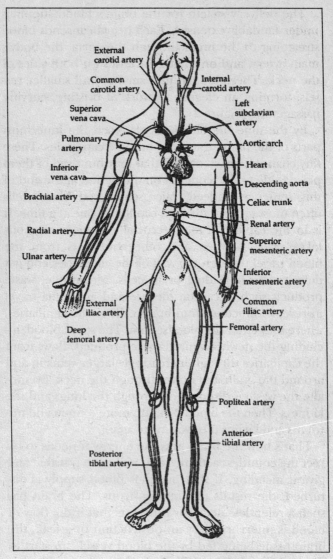

Figure 2. The circulatory system

function the affected neurons once served slips away, sometimes permanently. If a disrupted blood flow affects the very core of the brain—the part that keeps our lungs breathing and our heart pumping—a stroke can be fatal. As one eighteenth-century observer put it, a stroke can "utterly abolish the functions of the brain."

Fortunately, all strokes are not created equal. With severe strokes, patients may fall suddenly into a deep coma and be paralyzed. In less severe cases, patients may be fully conscious but may complain of numbness or weakness. Still others might feel dizzy or blurry-eyed for a short while before recovering with no aftereffects. Regardless of the symptoms, all strokes are serious emergencies that deserve prompt medical attention.

Let's review the types of strokes and explain which are most common in the black community—and why.

## TYPES OF STROKE

There are two major categories of stroke (Figures 3 and 4). About 85 percent of all strokes are classified as *ischemia* (is-ké-me-ah), also called *infarctions*. During an ischemic stroke, the normal flow of blood through the brain is blocked. The culprit is often a

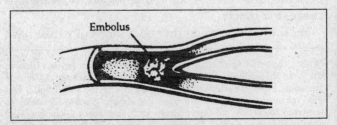

Figure 3. Ischemic stroke

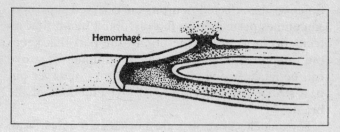

Figure 4. Hemorrhagic stroke

blood clot or a fatty deposit. In either case, brain tissue that lies "downstream" from the obstruction is denied life-giving nutrients.

The other 15 percent of strokes are some form of *hemorrhage*. With these, a blood vessel in the brain suddenly ruptures. Hemorrhagic strokes are caused by high blood pressure, among other things.* When delicate blood vessels can no longer contain highly pressurized blood, they burst like an overinflated inner tube. When that happens, blood that under normal circumstances is neatly contained inside arteries and veins leaks into the brain or surrounding tissues. There it disrupts the normal workings of neurons and puts pressure on crucial areas of the brain.

Thus ischemia and hemorrhage are very different—and in some ways opposite—problems. With ischemia, the brain gets too little blood. With hemorrhage, too much.

Yet there's one thing that both kinds of stroke have

---

*Other causes of hemorrhagic stroke include trauma (as in a blow to the head that ruptures a blood vessel); tumors; *arteriovenous* (AV) *malformation,* in which arteries and veins are connected in a fragile, tangled cluster with no intervening capillaries; *bleeding diathesis* (a tendency to bleed); substance abuse, including alcohol, cocaine, and amphetamines (Chapter 2); and anticoagulant therapy or *carotid endarterectomy* (Chapter 5).

in common: they are more prevalent—and more deadly—in the black community.

## Ischemic Strokes

There are three major types of ischemic stroke—the type of stroke caused by blocked blood vessels. They are TIA, thrombosis, and embolism.

*TIA or Mini-stroke*  The first type of stroke might not seem like a stroke at all, because it doesn't last for very long. It's called a *transient ischemic attack,* also called a TIA or "mini-stroke." In a typical case, a person may notice that the print in a telephone book looks blurry and one arm feels numb. But by the time they dial directory assistance, their vision is 20/20 again and their arm feels fine. Or someone may reach to shake the hand of a friend when suddenly part of their field of vision goes black and they can't verbalize the greeting they are thinking. Five minutes later, their eyesight is back and they are talking like normal.

A TIA is a sudden impairment of blood flow to the brain that typically lasts for less than a minute. The blockage is usually caused by a tiny blood clot or piece of debris from a fatty deposit in an artery. TIAs repair themselves when the obstruction dissolves, causing no permanent tissue damage and no lasting effects (Figure 5).

The symptoms vary. They depend on which artery happens to be blocked, and where along the blood vessel the blockage occurs. One of the more common scenarios is for a person to notice that their hand or foot has grown numb, or feels prickly or burning. The sensation then quickly spreads to the whole arm or leg or

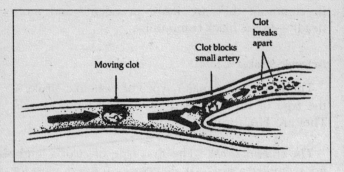

Figure 5. A transient ischemic attack (TIA)

to an entire side of the body before disappearing. Sometimes the person cannot see (or they see double) or speak (or they slur their words). They may feel dizzy or confused or have nausea or a headache. They may have a "drop attack"—falling to the floor without losing consciousness—because without warning their legs have become too weak to support them.

TIAs can be tricky to diagnose, because the symptoms can point to lots of disorders besides a stroke. It takes a skilled doctor to distinguish TIAs from other illnesses.

Sometimes TIAs are triggered by moderate or even mild exertion (for example, exercise, coughing, changes in posture, turning the head). Other times, they simply happen.

About 11 percent of all strokes are TIAs. In the general population, one person in a thousand suffers at least one TIA; among persons over age sixty-five, the rate triples to three in a thousand. TIAs are rarer in blacks than in whites.

TIA patients may suffer as few as several attacks over two or three years or as many as several in a day.

Regardless of how frequently they strike, the sad fact is that many patients simply brush them off. They chalk up the unusual symptoms to stress, or they reassure themselves that whatever happened must not be serious because the symptoms disappeared as suddenly as they came. But that's a big mistake. An estimated 35 to 50 percent of people who suffer a TIA and who seek no medical care suffer a crippling stroke within five years. Usually, the full-blown stroke occurs within a year of the TIA; in one reliable study, 24 percent of the subsequent strokes happened during the next *month*. In essence, TIAs function as an early warning. For those who heed the alarm, doctors can do a great deal to discover and correct the underlying problem. People who disregard the warning are taking a tremendous gamble.

If the symptoms of a transient attack last for more than a day, the event is classified as a full-fledged ischemic stroke. Ischemic strokes are caused by the gradual narrowing of an artery by fatty deposits, or the formation of a blood clot. This material plugs the bloodstream, preventing blood flow to the brain. There are two major types of ischemic stroke: *thrombosis* and *embolism** (Figure 6). The only difference between them is where the plug originates.

---

*There is also a third and less common form of ischemia known by the tongue-twister *hypoxic-ischemic encephalopathy*. Here the blood supply to the brain is impaired not by an obstruction in an artery, but by poor circulation to the entire body. For example, a person may have an erratic heartbeat or suffer a heart attack. Or a clot of blood or other material may become lodged in the pulmonary artery, which carries blood from the heart to the lungs—a life-threatening condition known as *pulmonary embolism*. Or a patient may be bleeding from somewhere in the stomach or intestines. Any of these conditions could cause the brain to receive an insufficient supply of blood.

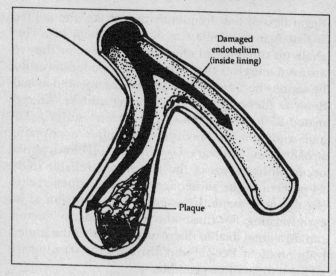

Figure 6.  Plaque build-up leading to thrombosis

*Thrombosis*  With thrombosis, a fatty deposit or a blood clot forms in one of the large arteries of the neck, or in blood vessels within and on the surface of the brain. Thrombosis is the most prevalent form of stroke, accounting for some 65 percent of all cases.

Thrombosis usually strikes when someone is sleeping or inactive for a period of time. A person will roll out of bed or stand from a chair only to find that one of their arms or legs shows a classic sign of stroke: weakness, numbness, or a prickling or burning sensation. Headache and seizures are not uncommon. These feelings worsen in stages over a period of anywhere from hours to months, with some improvement in the interim. If a patient has suffered a previous transient attack, the symptoms of the TIA will often mimic the thrombosis.

Thrombosis is most common in elderly patients whose arteries contain a buildup of yellowish fatty deposits called *plaque*. Researchers believe plaque deposits are caused by a number of factors, including diet, smoking, and high blood pressure. (We'll explain how in Chapter 2.) A typical thrombosis patient also has a history of diabetes or sickle cell anemia, both of which are prevalent among African-Americans.

One type of thrombosis that's particularly common in the black community is called a *lacunar stroke*. A *lacune* (lah-kune) is a small pit or cavity that can develop in the wall of a blood vessel, often as a result of chronic hypertension, which is prevalent among blacks. Hypertension frequently leads to *atherosclerosis,* or thickening and hardening of the arteries, in the minute blood vessels within the brain. Once these vessels become clogged with fatty debris, the blockage can do more than interrupt blood flow. It can also press on soft brain tissue. And when the fatty material eventually dissolves, the dent that remains in the tissue disturbs the proper functioning of the brain.

The onset of thrombosis is typically sudden, but lacunar strokes often get worse in stages. Over a period of one or two days, a patient who at first felt only mild weakness may eventually wind up completely paralyzed. Other common symptoms include mood fluctuations, headache, lightheadedness, hiccough, and a condition known as *asterixis*—the intermittent inability of the muscles to sustain someone's posture.

**Embolism**  An embolism (*embolus* is a Greek word for "plug") is similar to thrombosis, as noted above. But with an embolism, a fatty deposit or blood clot formed elsewhere in the body detaches and travels through increasingly narrow blood vessels, eventually becoming wedged in the neck or brain. There it can neither proceed further because of its size nor reverse course and travel upstream against the one-way blood flow. Embolisms cause about 10 percent of all strokes.

The blockage often originates in the large arteries that connect heart and brain. It can also come from a damaged heart in persons with rheumatic fever, *endocarditis* (inflammation of the membrane surrounding the heart), any of a number of heart-valve diseases, or in patients who have survived a heart attack or open-heart surgery. Embolism patients are often relatively young (fifty-six to sixty-four years old).

Unlike thrombosis, an embolism usually strikes when a person is active. The symptoms usually come on suddenly and may be minor and fleeting or major and permanent, depending on the size of the blockage and whether it is prone to break up once it has lodged in a blood vessel.

### Hemorrhagic Strokes

Human arteries are an engineering marvel. These long tubes—the pipes that carry blood from the heart to every corner of the body—are wrapped in a thin layer of muscle surrounded by a layer of elastic tissue. This combination of strength and elasticity pays off each time the heart beats. When the heart pumps, it sends a high-pressure surge of blood through the aorta, the body's largest artery. With each pulse, the aorta expands like a balloon (thanks to the elastic tissue) and contracts (because of muscle compression), which pushes the blood through the artery in a smooth ripple. The fact that the arteries can actually help pump blood helps the heart, which doesn't have to work as hard to ensure circulation.

But arteries have their limits. As a person's blood pressure climbs, the arteries become less elastic and less flexible, much like a garden hose stiffens when you open a faucet with the nozzle closed. Arteries also become more rigid as a person grows older. The combination of age and high pressure causes the arteries to lose their ability to flex to accommodate the surge of blood that follows each heartbeat. If the high blood pressure is not treated, it can eventually burst a blood vessel. The brain is a vulnerable location for this rupture because its delicate arteries and threadlike capillaries lack the thick muscles of the aorta.

Although African-Americans suffer all types of strokes, we are at high risk of hemorrhagic stroke because we are prone to hypertension. Dr. Edward S. Cooper of the University of Pennsylvania Hospital, an expert on stroke in blacks, goes so far as to call cerebral hemorrhage "the great killer in hypertensive blacks, especially young ones." Studies bear him out. Cooper cites research at Brooklyn's Kings County Hospital Center where, despite equivalent levels of high blood pressure, blacks suffered more "disastrous hemorrhagic complications" than did whites. Similarly, a Maryland study of 393 deaths from cerebral hemorrhage found that the average black patient was only forty-nine years old—twelve years younger than the average white patient.

There are two major types of hemorrhagic stroke: *cerebral* (also called *intracerebral*) and *subarachnoid*. Cerebral hemorrhage occurs inside the brain. In contrast, subarachnoid hemorrhage occurs between the surface of the brain and the inside of the skull. Cerebral hemorrhage is more common, accounting for about 10 percent of all stroke cases. Subarachnoid hemorrhage causes 5 percent of strokes.

Cerebral hemorrhage, usually caused by high blood pressure, can also result from an ischemic blood clot that presses on the walls of an artery where it is lodged, until the wall finally gives way. Occasionally, hemorrhagic strokes are caused by an *aneurism* (an´-yur-ism)—a weak area that forms a bulge in the arterial wall owing to the pressure of blood flowing through the artery (Figure 7). Aneurisms are often harmless; people can live with them for their whole lives without any problems. But if an aneurism bursts—or if a blood vessel ruptures for any reason— the effects of the hemorrhage are often catastrophic. At the site of the hemorrhage, blood streams from the open artery and into the folds and crevices of brain matter. The bleeding puts extreme pressure on nearby brain tissue and sometimes even displaces it. It may not be surprising, then, that in about half of all

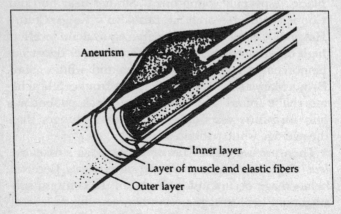

Figure 7. An aneurism

patients, the first sign of cerebral hemorrhage is a sudden intense headache. Victims may experience nausea or vomiting, become delirious, or lose consciousness. Within a few hours or a few days, the stroke can bring anything from paralysis to coma to death, depending on where the rupture occurs.

In contrast to cerebral hemorrhage, which occurs within the brain, subarachnoid hemorrhages bleed into the so-called subarachnoid space—a fluid-filled area of delicate tissue ("arachnoid" is Greek for "like a spider's web") that surrounds the brain. Blood leaking into the subarachnoid space becomes trapped within the bony confines of the skull, and puts excruciating pressure on soft and fragile brain tissue. Often the cause is an aneurism that may vary from the size of a matchtip to the size of a strawberry. In fact, some of these bulges are called "berry aneurisms" because of their shape.

Subarachnoid hemorrhage is most common in persons age twenty-five to fifty, and blacks seem to be at greater risk than whites. This type of stroke often comes on during physical exertion (lifting, bending, straining). The patient is typically hit with a severe headache, fever, vision problems, or facial or neck pain and over time may become confused or dazed. People usually survive their first attack, but additional bleeding sometimes follows within days or a few weeks.

Sometimes subarachnoid hemorrhages send subtle signals—chronic neck pain, or nausea, or headache. Unfortunately, these warning signs are frequently misunderstood. "Many patients arrive at the neurosurgeon's doorstep too ill to be saved," writes Dr. Louis R. Caplan, chairman of the Department of

Neurology at Tufts University School of Medicine and the New England Medical Center in Boston. "Either the patient had not sought medical advice or physicians had missed the significance of the symptoms of headache, vomiting, or inability to function."

## BRINGING IT ALL TOGETHER

The word "stroke" usually brings to mind an elderly person who cannot speak or is partially paralyzed. In reality, as we've seen, a stroke can mean many different things. Most strokes affect the elderly, but some (especially in the black community) strike young or middle-aged adults. Some strokes cause paralysis and loss of speech. Others cause any number of disorders, from collapse to coma to confusion. Some strokes happen suddenly. Others send warnings. Some strokes are devastating, causing permanent and massive damage. Others come gently, causing subtle effects that disappear within a few seconds.

Despite these differences, strokes have certain elements in common. First, no stroke is trivial. It stands to reason that any illness that leaves a person unable to use their arms or legs, or that robs them of their vision or speech, is a serious medical emergency. But even when the symptoms are relatively minor and short-lived, strokes mean brain damage. Anyone who suffers the symptoms of a stroke should seek medical care immediately.

Second, many strokes are preventable. Living a healthful lifestyle—controlling blood pressure, maintaining appropriate weight, exercising regularly—can greatly reduce the risk of ever suffering a stroke. We'll find out more about how to boost your chances of avoiding a stroke in Chapter 5.

For people who suffer a "mini-stroke" or TIA—a warning sign of a more serious stroke—and seek prompt medical care, doctors can do a great deal to prevent a full-fledged stroke from occurring. We'll learn more about treating stroke in Chapter 3.

# CHAPTER 2

# Black Folks at Risk

Iran-Contra, junk bonds making other folks rich, and ketchup dressed up as a vegetable. That's what the 1980s meant to million of African-Americans.

But if you ask Joe Williams* what the "me decade" meant to him, he'll tell you break dancing. One New Year's Eve, Williams did what many partygoers do to celebrate the passage of another year: he put away a few drinks and got a little wild. He had seen others break-dance but he had never tried it himself, so he headed for the dance floor.

When Joe Williams woke the next morning, his head was pounding. But this was no routine hangover: he was also partially blind. Doctors administered a CT-scan only to discover that a blood vessel inside his head had burst, and he was bleeding into his brain. The twenty-seven-year-old had suffered a stroke. Fortunately, the hemorrhage eventually healed and his headache and blindness disappeared.

Joe's doctors, who had never before seen such a

---

*Not his real name.

thing, guessed that the combination of alcohol and the violent head movements had caused too much strain on the fragile blood vessels inside his head. They were so alarmed that they wrote a letter to the *New England Journal of Medicine:* "In view of the potential hazards, we advise caution for those who want to break dance, especially while under the influence of alcohol."

Good advice? Maybe not. Young Williams had none of the medical conditions that predispose a person to stroke. He was young, not elderly. His blood pressure was normal, not high. And he denied taking street drugs, which can raise blood pressure. His stroke was clearly a fluke, a once-in-a-million event. If every person who tried to break-dance ended up in a hospital emergency room with a stroke, people would avoid it like the plague. But they don't, because the probability of getting a stroke from break dancing is remote.

Medicine is about probability. If your appendix is inflamed, taking it out usually leads to complete recovery. If you are tense, a quiet walk around the block will often help you relax. If your blood pressure is high, following your doctor's advice will usually lower it.

Researchers have spent many years and countless dollars to understand the workings of stroke, and the medical breakthroughs in the past decade or two alone have been eye-opening. One of the questions scientists are answering is why stroke is more likely to strike certain people. When researchers talk about the probability that someone will contract a disease, they use the term "risk factor." A risk factor is a condition that increases a person's chance of getting sick.

## RISK FACTORS

### Types of Risk Factors

There are many ways of thinking about risk factors. Some risk factors are physiological, having to do with the makeup of our bodies. For example, diabetes runs in the family. If your parent or uncle or grandmother had diabetes, your chances of having it are increased compared to someone without a family history of the disease. Another example is heart disease, which strikes men more often than it does women. Hip fractures affect senior citizens more than they do teenagers. Physiological risk factors are not preventable because they are a part of who we are. We can't change our genes, our gender, or our age (although a health-conscious lifestyle and regular medical care can help prevent medical problems or help heal them if they develop).

In contrast, other risk factors have more to do with our environment. For instance, the risk of developing cirrhosis, the liver disease, can be reduced dramatically by not abusing alcohol. The nicotine addiction that hooks people on cigarettes can be successfully treated with hypnosis, group therapy, or special smoking-withdrawal clinics. These types of risk factors are caused by our lifestyles and our surroundings. These risk factors are preventable.

Many diseases have both physiological and environmental risk factors. Stroke is a prime example. Researchers have identified nearly two dozen risk factors for stroke. Some (race, age, heredity) we can do little about. Others (cigarette smoking, use of oral contraceptives) we can control. Certain risk factors for stroke are themselves the products of both physiological and environmental conditions. Heart disease is a good example. Some people are prone to heart disease because they are obese—a condition that may be imbedded in the family's genes (a physiological risk factor) as well as in eating habits (an environmental risk factor).

### How strong is the evidence?

The strength of the scientific evidence that links each risk factor to stroke varies. Some risk factors are infamous, having been chronicled for many years. For example, the first meaningful account of stroke was recorded in the late fifth century B.C. by the Greek physician Hippocrates. He wrote that "persons are most subject to apoplexy [stroke] between the ages of forty and sixty." At a time when few people lived to see their sixtieth birthday, Hippocrates had discovered a key risk factor for stroke: old age. Other well-established risk factors include hypertension, heart disease, and either having suffered a stroke or having relatives who have.

In contrast, some risk factors for stroke are backed by weaker evidence. In these cases, scientists may not have conducted definitive studies, or the studies might have yielded conflicting results, or it may otherwise be difficult to tie the risk factor to the disease. Using oral contraceptives is a weak risk factor for stroke, as is a certain type of obesity.

### Is it important?

If the evidence behind a risk factor is strong, doctors usually focus on it as an important predictor of disease or illness. With stroke, two prime examples are old age and hypertension. Both are backed by years of study, and both are key concerns when a physician evaluates a person's potential for stroke. There are exceptions, however. A narrowing of the neck arteries—a condition marked by an audible sign called a *bruit* [broo´-it or brew´-ee]—is a well-established risk factor for stroke. But physicians, particularly those in the black community, tend not to focus on it as much as they concentrate on hypertension and other major risk factors that are hitting African-Americans left and right. It's a matter of priorities, and not every risk factor deserves the same weight, even when the evidence implicating it is reliable.

### Can it be treated?

Finally, some risk factors can be treated more effectively than others. Hypertension is a classic treatable risk factor. It can be controlled with medicine, diet, stress reduction, or a combination of the three. For other risk factors, researchers either haven't yet devised effective treatments, or they haven't determined that treating a condition causes any real reduction in stroke risk.

What, then, have we learned about risk factors? Environmental risk factors are preventable; physiological ones are not. Some risk factors are well established; others are suggestive. Some risk factors are more important than others. And some are more treatable than others. Let's take a closer look at some of the risk factors for stroke, and then turn our attention to why African-Americans are especially vulnerable.

**1. Age**
   **Type of risk factor:** Nonpreventable
   **Strength of evidence:** Well established
   **Treatment:** Not feasible
   **Importance:** Major

You don't have to be elderly to have a stroke. A fair number of stroke patients are under the age of sixty-five, and some of them aren't even adults. Strokes in newborn babies are a major cause of cerebral palsy, and African-Americans with sickle cell anemia often suffer strokes in childhood.

But the risk of suffering a stroke increases dramatically as people get older. In fact, the chances of having a stroke double for every decade that a person lives over the age of fifty-five. About 80 percent of strokes occur in people over the age of sixty-five, and 90 percent happen in those over the age of fifty-five. These statistics have a direct bearing on the African-American community, because our population is growing twice as fast as the white population. And that means that each year, as more and more black people age, the number of blacks at risk of stroke increases.

Why do older people suffer more strokes? One theory is that advancing years cause a breakdown in *collagen*, a protein that forms much of the connective tissue in the body. A breakdown of the collagen in skin cells explains why skin wrinkles and sags as we get older. Collagen is also what gives blood vessels their strength. So when collagen begins to break down, the blood vessel wall loses its holding power, much like a paper bag does when wet.

In addition, old age frequently brings on hypertension. The two numbers used to measure blood pressure reflect how high (in millimeters) the heart would push a column of mercury during *systole* (sis´-tuh-lee), or contraction of the heart, and *diastole* (die-ass´-tuh-lee), or relaxation of the heart. Systolic pressure (the higher number) tends to increase bit by bit as we get older, at least in women. Diastolic pressure rises during the early adult years but often levels off when a person is in their fifties and sixties, after which it sometimes declines.

We'll take a closer look at hypertension below. For now, suffice it to say that unchecked high blood pressure in an elderly person is too dangerous to ignore. When you imagine what happens when increasingly pressurized blood pushes against age-weakened blood vessels, it's not difficult to see why doctors say the most important uncontrollable risk factor for stroke is age.

2. **Hypertension (high blood pressure)**
   **Type of risk factor:** Preventable and nonpreventable aspects
   **Strength of evidence:** Well established
   **Treatment:** Possible
   **Importance:** Major

High blood pressure is much more common among blacks than it is among whites. In fact, hypertension is so prevalent in the black community that it's easy to take it for granted. Many African-American youngsters grow up hearing someone—a grandparent, a church elder, a neighbor—talk about their "pressure." Many of us may assume that high blood pressure is an inevitable part of growing old. It isn't. But one thing *is* for certain: *untreated* hypertension is an open invitation for stroke. Dr. Edward S. Cooper is blunt on the subject. "Hypertension is definitely the main underlying risk factor and cause of stroke," says Dr. Cooper. "Adequate control of mild, moderate, and severe hypertension will prevent most strokes, especially in blacks." As a matter of fact, the overall United States death rate from stroke has dropped 50 percent in the last fifteen years, and the death rate in the black community has fallen even more. Most experts credit better control of hypertension.

Hypertension greatly increases the risk of both ischemic and hemorrhagic stroke. "Indeed," says Dr. Charles K. Francis of the Harlem Hospital Center, "we often say that we do not treat hypertension because high blood pressure is dangerous; we treat hypertension because strokes and coronary [heart] disease are dangerous." When blood is under sufficiently high pressure, it can literally burst through the wall of a cerebral artery. The brain's arteries come equipped with a remarkable defense mechanism: they squeeze as a person's blood pressure increases. This helps contain the increasingly pressurized blood and helps ensure a normal supply of blood to all-important brain tissues. In cases of severe hypertension, however, a person's blood pressure climbs so high that this self-regulating mechanism is overwhelmed. This is when the balloonlike swelling of a blood vessel can lead to hemorrhagic stroke.

There's a second way that hypertension can cause a stroke. Hypertension seems to accelerate atherosclerosis—the thickening and narrowing of the arteries by fatty plaque. The mechanism for this hazardous transformation has do with collagen, the tough protein that gives bones, skin, and cartilage their strength. Healthy arteries are lined with a protective layer of *endothelial* (en´-do-thee´-lee-all) cells. Collagen lies underneath these cells. In the arteries of a person with hypertension, the high blood pressure damages the endothelial layer, exposing collagen to the bloodstream. When this happens, the collagen attracts *platelets*—blood cells responsible for clotting—and causes them to stick together and to secrete a chemical that induces more platelets, plus fibrous tissue, bloodstream debris, and cholesterol from the blood, to clump together as well. The chain reaction eventually results in the accumulation of fatty material inside the arterial wall, where it thickens and narrows the artery (Figure 8).

This can cause even more hypertension, because the same amount of blood must now squeeze into a smaller space. What's more, a thickened artery loses the elasticity it needs to expand and contract with each heartbeat, which means the shock of each pulse is no longer dampened. If the artery is eventually blocked by the fatty deposit (or a piece of it that detaches), the end result can be an ischemic stroke. If the blockage causes the blood vessel to break open, the result is a hemorrhagic stroke.

This risk is very real. People who have borderline hypertension (blood pressure between 140/90 and 160/95) are twice as likely to have a stroke than are so-called normotensives—people with normal blood pressure (under 140/90). Persons with definite hypertension (blood pressure higher than 160/95) are four times as likely. And in one analysis of patients by the Framingham (Massachusetts) Heart Study, one of the nation's most influential and longest-running heart studies, the risk of ischemic stroke in patients with hypertension was higher than the risk in normotensives by a factor of seven.

Researchers don't know all the reasons why hypertension is more prevalent in the black community, but they have some important clues. Hypertension may be somehow related to skin color; studies show that darker-skinned blacks have higher blood pressure than do blacks with lighter skin, perhaps because darker-skinned African-Americans face harsher racism. Hypertension may also be genetic, with the traits for the disorder being passed in the black community from generation to generation.

How do your genes affect your blood pressure? One theory is that the ability to retain sodium helped slaves survive inhuman living conditions during passage to America, when food and water were scarce, and diarrhea and seasickness depleted slaves of nutrients. Dr. Clarence Grim, at the Charles Drew/UCLA Hypertension Research Center in Los Angeles, thinks that the slaves whose bodies could hoard salt survived and passed on this genetic trait to future generations. Regrettably, while the typical diet of today's African-Americans is awash in too much sodium, our genes are still programmed to conserve it. And that creates problems, because too much sodium is a major cause of hypertension. Sodium is important for the human

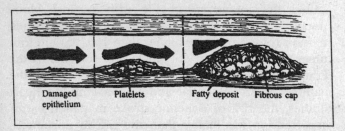

Damaged          Platelets          Fatty deposit    Fibrous cap
epithelium

Figure 8.  Formation of plaque

body; everyone needs a little to function normally. But we only need a tiny amount. In larger doses. it acts like a poison. When we eat too much of it, our bodies automatically retain fluids to dilute the sodium down to a safe level. These same fluids collect in the bloodstream, where they eventually cause high blood pressure.

Sodium isn't the only dietary villain. The cholesterol and fat in our food affects our blood pressure, too. When we eat too much rich, greasy food, our bodies can't digest all of the extra fat and cholesterol. The extra winds up circulating in our bloodstream, where it attaches to the inside wall of arteries. That's the beginning of atherosclerosis, which, as we've seen above, raises the blood pressure.

Finally, hypertension is more common in the black community because of our environment. Blacks are typically under more stress than are whites. Studies show that your blood pressure rises while you're being subjected to the stress; when the stress lets up, blood pressure usually diminishes. But over time, repeated exposure to stressful situations can raise your blood pressure permanently. One Detroit study compared the blood pressure of whites and blacks living in high-stress areas (areas with lots of poverty, crowded housing, crime, marriage breakups, etc.) with whites and blacks living in low-stress areas. The people found to have the highest blood pressures—and perhaps not coincidentally, the highest levels of suppressed hostility—were black men in high-stress areas.

## 3. Heart disease
**Type of risk factor:** Preventable and nonpreventable aspects

**Strength of evidence:** Well established
**Treatment:** Possible
**Importance:** Major

Three out of four stroke patients have some form of heart disease. "Heart disease" covers a lot of territory, because the list of disorders that interfere with the normal workings of the heart is long. Heart disease can affect the heart's nerves or muscle. It can even affect the heart's valves, the tiny gateways that open and shut to keep blood flowing in one direction (Figure 9).

For years, many people assumed that heart disease mainly affected white people. That may have been true at one time, but not anymore. Today, African-Americans have about the same risk of developing heart problems as do whites. Black women, in fact, are more likely to have heart attacks—the most common form of heart disease—than are white women.

People who have heart disease frequently have hypertension as well, and it is often difficult to tell which of the two conditions makes them more prone to stroke. Nevertheless, evidence implicating certain heart diseases does exist. For example, *mitral valve prolapse*, in which one of the heart's valves fails to make a tight seal with surrounding tissue, appears to slightly increase the risk of ischemic stroke, possibly because the condition can give rise to clots. Coronary artery disease, the thickening and narrowing of the arteries that serve the heart, is also tied to ischemia, mainly by the same disease (atherosclerosis) that clogs other arteries. Other heart diseases that predispose a person for stroke include congestive heart failure; enlargement of the heart, which can be seen by X ray or electrocardiogram (ECG or EKG); and *atrial fibrillation,* an abnormal twitching of the heart chamber that receives blood from the veins. All in all, persons with impaired hearts have twice the risk of stroke than do persons with normal hearts.

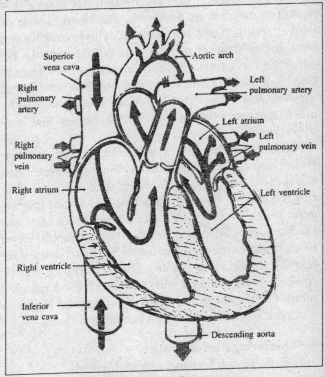

Figure 9. Valves inside the heart

Finally, there's a condition called *left ventricular hypertrophy*. This enlargement of the left side of the heart may triple a person's risk of stroke. Dr. William Castelli, director of the Framingham Heart Study, says that the size of the left ventricle—the pumping chamber that pushes blood into the aorta and throughout the body—is the price people pay for being overweight or having high blood pressure. "It's as powerful [a risk factor] as cholesterol, blood pressure, and smoking," says Dr. Castelli. "It means that person is headed in a big way for heart attack or stroke." Fortunately, left ventricular hypertrophy can be a doctor's tip-off to intervene before a stroke occurs. "We can't treat left ventricular mass," Dr. Jerome Cohen of the St. Louis University Medical School told the *New York Times*. "But [when we spot it] we can be more aggressive about looking for factors that contribute to it."

Heart disease is one of the few risk factors whose *cure* occasionally causes a stroke. Persons whose heart valves must be surgically replaced with artificial valves run the risk of developing a blood clot that can migrate to the brain. In fact, strokes can occur after any cardiac surgery. Despite these risks, you should never hesitate to get medical treatment for heart disease for fear of suffering a stroke. The chances of having stroke can be reduced with proper medical management. Compared to the harm of unchecked heart disease, the risk of stroke is much smaller indeed.

> **4. Suffering a prior stroke**
> **Type of risk factor:** Preventable and
> nonpreventable aspects
> **Strength of evidence:** Well established
> **Treatment:** Value not established
> **Importance:** Major

If an illness that's *related* to stroke (like heart disease) can make a person more prone to suffer a stroke, then you can understand why an actual stroke makes a person more likely to have another. If you have a stroke, your chances of having a second stroke are anywhere from ten to twenty times higher than the risk to a person who's never had a stroke at all. For blacks, this translates to perhaps a 15 to 20 percent chance of a second stroke—about the same as for whites—in the year following a full-blown ischemic stroke. After a TIA, the chances of being hit with a full ischemic stroke are even higher—up to 50 percent. The odds for second hemorrhagic strokes haven't been studied.

If a stroke has already occurred, it may seem too late to step in with preventive measures. But many stroke patients are neither killed nor permanently disabled. For these survivors, aggressive action to prevent a more serious stroke makes a good deal of sense.

### 5. Diabetes
**Type of risk factor:** Preventable and nonpreventable aspects
**Strength of evidence:** Well established
**Treatment:** Value not established for stroke
**Importance:** Major

In some hospitals, as many as 30 percent of the persons admitted for ischemic stroke have diabetes. Indeed, diabetics are six times more likely than others to suffer a stroke. One reason is that diabetics have a high incidence of diseases such as atherosclerosis; compared to nondiabetics, their arteries become thick with fatty deposits more often, earlier in life, and with greater severity. Nevertheless, research from the Framingham Heart Study indicates that diabetics who are otherwise healthy and who lack preexisting disorders have about the same low risk of stroke as do persons without diabetes. In other words, if you stay healthy and keep your diabetes under control, you probably won't have to worry about having a stroke.

Diabetes was rare in the black community until the twentieth century. Today it is a leading killer of blacks. Of thirty million African-Americans, there are an estimated two million diabetics, half of them undiagnosed—a rate 91 percent higher in blacks than in whites. And the prevalence of diabetes starts to climb as people age; among the sixty-five- to seventy-four-year-old age group, one in four African-Americans has diabetes.

The tendency to develop diabetes is carried in a person's genes, so in one sense the risk factor is unavoidable. But blacks and others who are prone to the disease can do a great deal to minimize the risk, including getting regular medical care, following a doctor's advice, eating prudently, and exercising regularly. Weight control is very important for black diabetics, most of whom are obese and have Type 2 diabetes—a form of the disease that often clears up entirely when a diabetic returns to normal weight. That's why diabetes as a risk factor involves both preventable and nonpreventable aspects.

Although the health risk from diabetes itself declines as people take better care of themselves, there's no clear evidence that treating diabetes lessens the risk of having a stroke. But that doesn't mean diabetics should ignore their disease. If you're diabetic and you happen to have a stroke when your blood sugar is high, there's strong evidence that any brain damage will be much more serious than if your blood sugar is low. That's only one reason that diabetics should follow their doctor's advice about diet, medication, and exercise. There are many other reasons, of course: diabetics who control their disease lead longer, more productive, more enjoyable lives.

**6. Smoking**
   **Type of risk factor:** Preventable
   **Strength of evidence:** Well established
   **Treatment:** Possible
   **Importance:** Major

Cigarette smoking has been called one of the greatest public health menaces in the world. To all of the many reasons not to smoke—bronchitis, emphysema, lung cancer, heart disease—should we add stroke? Not too long ago, doctors didn't think so. Some studies had found no link between smoking and stroke— or even an inverse risk, meaning that smokers had fewer strokes than did nonsmokers. But the tide began to turn in 1967, when a study of fifty thousand former students at two New England colleges found that students who smoked were twice as likely as non-smokers to have a fatal ischemic stroke later in life. Then the Framingham Heart Study found smoking to be a definite risk factor for ischemia in men under the age of sixty-five. In 1984, the American Heart Association added smoking to its list of possible risk factors for stroke.

Four years later came the most solid evidence to date. From the Boston University Medical Center came the results of a study that followed 4,255 men and women for twenty-six years. Smoking was a significant risk factor for stroke, especially for women smokers, and people who smoked two packs of cigarettes a day were at twice the risk of stroke than were people who smoked half a pack.

The links between smoking and stroke are the latest in a string of warning signs for African-American smokers. But more of us—black men, especially—need to listen. About 34 percent of black men smoke, compared to 28 percent of white men, 25 percent of white women, and 21 percent of black women. Black youth get lots of bad press, but on tobacco they're really ahead of the pack. From 1976 to 1996 the percentage of high school seniors who smoke fell 9 percent for whites but a whopping 74 percent for blacks. As black folks we're often advised to hear to the wisdom of our elders; here's a case where we could all take a lesson from our kids.

Researchers do have encouraging news for smokers as well: the many benefits of not smoking begin to accrue almost immediately after you kick the habit. Once a person quits smoking the risk of having a stroke begins to fall within months, according to Boston University scientists. By the end of two years quitters enjoy a substantial health advantage over people who continue to smoke. The researchers called their findings about quitters "quite favorable for the substantial number of middle-aged and elderly persons who have been long-term cigarette smokers."

**7. Alcohol consumption**
   **Type of risk factor:** Preventable
   **Strength of evidence:** Reasonably well established
   **Treatment:** Value not established
   **Importance:** Moderate

Alcohol—particularly in large amounts—has never been kind to the human body. In addition to cirrhosis and nerve damage in adults, and permanent birth defects in infants whose mothers drink alcohol, excessive alcohol consumption seems to heighten the risk for stroke. When does drinking become excessive? There are certainly some people who are so sensitive to alcohol that a few sips make them intoxicated. But to increase a person's risk of stroke, the danger level seems to be around three alcoholic drinks a day. When physicians at Kaiser Permanente Medical Care Program in Oakland, California, surveyed over one hundred thousand patients participating in a prepaid health plan, people who downed more than three drinks (wine, beer, or hard liquor) per day were up to four times more likely than abstainers to have a hemorrhagic stroke. The researchers felt that alcohol contributed to either hypertension or a tendency to bleed.

Like smoking, alcohol consumption is controllable, and alcoholism can be treated.

8. **Relatives who suffer a stroke**
   **Type of risk factor:** Preventable and
   nonpreventable aspects
   **Strength of evidence:** Well established
   **Treatment:** Variable
   **Importance:** Moderate

Stroke casts a broad net. Like other diseases that run in the family, this one spreads risk factors among relatives. For example, studies show that the parents of a stroke patient are at higher-than-usual risk of stroke themselves. The converse is also true, at least for mothers: if a mother has died of a stroke or suffered a series of TIAs, her children have an increased risk of stroke. Oddly, this relationship is not as strong among fathers and children; no one knows why. The National Institutes of Health says that as risk factors go, having a mother who died of stroke is not as significant as having heart disease, high blood pressure, or any of the more classic risk factors for stroke.

Family history is an unusual risk factor. In one sense, a family's medical history is beyond any one person's control; babies don't choose the family they are born into. So if your mother died of a stroke, you can't change that. But if her stroke was caused by hypertension or heart disease, you can certainly take steps to control those diseases in your own life. So to the extent that family history points to health problems that we can influence, a relative's illness may indicate a controllable risk factor for ourselves.

### 9. Gender
**Type of risk factor:** Nonpreventable
**Strength of evidence:** Well established
**Treatment:** Not possible
**Importance:** Moderate

Sixty percent of all stroke deaths involve women, which at first might lead you to think that women are at higher risk. Actually, the opposite is true. Men have more risk factors; they have higher blood pressure, they have more heart disease, and they smoke more cigarettes. All in all, men have 20 percent more strokes than do women. Women die more often simply because they live longer, so that by old age there are more of them who *can* be stroke patients. That's why the death rate from stroke is higher in women (around 96,000 stroke deaths in 1995) than in men (62,000 stroke deaths).

Researchers have suspected for years that estrogen, the female sex hormone, helps protect women from stroke. A recent study at a California retirement community confirmed the value of estrogen supplements in preventing strokes in older women. Unfortunately, though men's bodies naturally contain traces of the female hormone, estrogen supplements don't do men much good. Research shows that men have just as many strokes whether they're taking estrogen tablets or not. For now, the reason men have a higher stroke risk than women remains a mystery. Researchers do know, however, that men and women tend to have different *types* of stroke. Men have more ischemic strokes than do women; women have more subarachnoid hemorrhage than do men.

### 10. Obesity
**Type of risk factor:** Preventable and nonpreventable aspects
**Strength of evidence:** Variable depending on type of obesity
**Treatment:** Possible but value not established
**Importance:** Variable

Doctors define obesity as 20 percent or more over a person's ideal body weight. Obesity can be a major risk factor for stroke, but the degree of risk depends on where the excess weight is distributed. According to the National Institutes of Health, men who have "beer bellies" or "spare tires" are at significant risk for stroke. Other forms of obesity appear to be related to stroke, too, but not because of obesity itself: overweight people in general frequently have high blood pressure or diabetes, two risk factors for stroke. That's especially true for African-Americans, who are more obese than whites and who also have more hypertension and diabetes. For adults age twenty to seventy-four, the prevalence of obesity is similar in white men (59 percent) and black men (58 percent), but there's a substantial difference between the obesity rate for white women (45 percent) and black women (66 percent).

## 11. Bruits

**Type of risk factor:** Nonpreventable
**Strength of evidence:** Well established
**Treatment:** Value not established
**Importance:** Limited

Many risk factors for stroke are conditions that a physician can see. A bruit is a risk factor that a doctor can hear.

A bruit is the sound that blood makes when it changes speed and direction as it streams through a narrowed blood vessel. Through a stethoscope, a bruit may have any number of sounds, including a soft high-pitched murmur or the sound of water lapping the shore of a lake. Each sound signals a different type of obstruction inside the artery. When doctors examine you to evaluate your risk for stroke, they may listen for bruits in blood vessels between the heart and the head. They will pay special attention to the carotid, a major neck artery that is prone to blockage in persons with atherosclerosis.

Bruits are called asymptomatic when they cause no discomfort or other ill effects. But research suggests that even persons with asymptomatic bruits are at risk for later stroke. One study in Evans County, Georgia, which is about 40 percent black, found that of 1,620 people surveyed, 72 had bruits. Within six years, 10 of the 72 (13.0 percent) had suffered a stroke. In contrast, only 3.4 percent of the people without bruits had had a stroke.

On the other hand, strokes often occur far away from the site of a bruit—and frequently on the opposite side of the body entirely. And sometimes the strokes are caused by aneurisms or blood clots from the heart—two causes that have nothing to do with a bruit. For these reasons, doctors say that a bruit isn't a fool-proof indicator.

Researchers do agree that bruits increase a person's risk of dying of stroke by nearly a factor of two. On average, 3 to 4 percent of the population over the age of forty-five have bruits, and the prevalence increases with age. Treatment—surgically removing the blockage—is risky and expensive; the complication rate in the 1984 Toronto Asymptomatic Prospective Cervical Bruit Study ("cervical" refers to the neck) was an uncomfortable 16.7 percent. But although the value of treatment is disputable, the value of identifying persons with bruits is not: a person with a bruit may have other risk factors that can be controlled.

12. **Cocaine use**
    **Type of risk factor:** Preventable
    **Strength of evidence:** Recent but strong
    **Treatment:** Possible
    **Importance:** High for cocaine users

A young man reaches for a crack pipe, searching for euphoria. What he actually gets is a tragedy: paralysis from a stroke. It's a scene that's repeated so frequently in hospitals across the country that doctors are revising their checklist of what to look for when they examine emergency room patients. A decade ago, no one expected a young hospital patient who had difficulty speaking or walking to have suffered a drug-induced stroke. Then again, ten years ago, no one understood the grim legacy of cocaine.

Once it is snorted, injected, or smoked, cocaine causes a number of alarming effects. The heartbeat accelerates. Blood pressure shoots up. Blood vessels squeeze tight. The sudden burst in blood pressure might cause a stroke by hemorrhage; if the arteries being squeezed are located in the brain, ischemic stroke might result when the brain receives insufficient oxygen.

Cocaine is particularly cruel to the unborn child. A mother who uses cocaine, even briefly, risks giving her infant a multitude of problems, including prematurity or low birthweight; behavioral abnormalities such as extreme irritability and inability to be consoled; and physical abnormalities ranging from malformed organs to a missing small intestine. In extreme cases, the sudden increase in blood pressure gives the unborn child a stroke. What happens then? Dr. Ira Chasnoff, director of Northwestern University's Perinatal Center for Chemical Dependence, tells of a suburban woman whose husband gave her five grams of cocaine as an anniversary gift. She had given up the drug during her pregnancy, but the gift proved too tempting to pass up. In the mother's womb, the child had a stroke that damaged a significant portion of his brain. He was born like so many thousands of stroke patients many decades his senior—unable to fully use his right arm and leg.

Strokes have been linked to other drugs besides cocaine.

---

### Drug Abuse and Stroke

If you love sports and you have a good memory, you may remember the tragic story of Len Bias, the rising basketball star for the Boston Celtics. Bias's 1986 death from cocaine-induced heart failure brought home for all of us the cardiovascular dangers of cocaine. But as Americans mourned another drug casualty, probably few realized that cocaine can also cause strokes.

In fact, a number of drugs have been linked with stroke. Cocaine is perhaps the most publicized, but amphetamines and similar stimulants have been linked to both cerebral and subarachnoid hemorrhage, often in habitual abusers but sometimes in first-time users. Drugs in this class include PPA (phenylpropanolamine), an ingredient in over-the-counter diet aids such as Dexatrim and Prolamine, and pseudoephedrine, a popularr decongestant found in Contac, Sine-Aid, and similar products. The potential for stroke comes from these medicines' ability to increase blood pressure. While most persons who use these products according to the manufacturer's recommendations suffer few dangerous side effects, those who abuse the drugs by exceeding the suggested doses can run into problems. Sensitive persons may experience trouble even after abiding by the manufacturer's recommended dosages.

Likewise, PCP (phencyclidine or "angel dust") and LSD, both of which elevate blood pressure, have been known to cause hemorrhagic strokes in persons as young as six years old, and barbiturates and other tranquilizers and sedatives have caused ischemic stroke in some drug abusers.

Many of the dozens who have suffered drug-induced strokes have died within a matter of days, their brains too compromised to carry out even the most basic functions.

---

## 13. Blood disorders

Five blood disorders are risk factors for stroke. Medical treatment can reduce the risk for at least two of them. With the exception of sickle cell anemia, these blood disorders are rare. In most cases, you probably wouldn't know you had one unless a doctor told you. So don't lose sleep over these blood disorders. For any given person, chances are the more infamous risk factors for stroke—high blood pressure, heart disease, prior stroke—are much more inportant.

**a. Sickle cell anemia**
   **Type of risk factor:** Nonpreventable
   **Strength of evidence:** Well established
   **Treatment:** Possible
   **Importance:** Major in the black community

Sickle cell anemia affects over fifty thousand black Americans—8 percent of our community—with an array of debilitating health problems, including stroke. Sickle cell anemia affects the structure of hemoglobin, the iron-carrying molecule in red blood cells. The disease makes normally separate hemoglobin molecules join together in long strands. This one small alteration affects the shape of up to 40 percent of the patient's red blood cells (Figure 10). Normal red cells are gently rounded disks with a flattened center. Sickled blood cells look like an elongated letter "c," four or five times as long from tip to tip as a normal cell is wide. Sickle cell patients have so many of these abnormal cells that they overtax the spleen, whose job is to remove old or damaged red blood cells. Eventually, so many red blood cells are removed from circulation that the remainder cannot carry enough oxygen throughout the body, and the result is anemia.

The disease puts people at risk of stroke in two ways.

First, sickled cells can get stuck in slender capillaries, which, you may recall, are often only wide enough to permit passage of one normal-sized red blood cell at a time. But there's an even greater threat. For some reason, the arteries leading to the brain of sickle cell patients can become narrowed through a buildup of scar tissue. This in turn increases the likelihood that sickled cells will accumulate and, like cars in a traffic pile-up, eventually block the flow of blood to the brain.

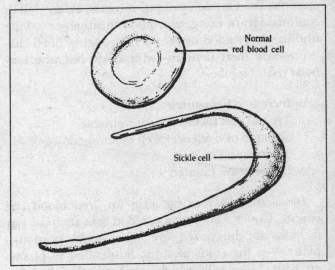

Figure 10. Sickle cell anemia

Up to 17 percent of all sickle cell patients have strokes, most of them around the tender age of ten. In fact, stroke accounts for 16 percent of childhood deaths from sickle cell anemia.

There is no cure for sickle cell anemia, but a recently developed ultrasound test is a promising way to identify sickle cell patients at highest risk for stroke.

Once doctors find the disorder, they can treat it and prevent some of its more serious complications. One exciting treatment option is giving blood transfusions. In a 1997 study sponsored by the National Institutes of Health, blood transfusions given every three to four weeks to children with sickle cell anemia cut their risk of stroke by an amazing 90 percent. The study was so successful that it was halted sixteen months earlier than planned; the scientists had seen enough. Dr. Claude Lenfant, director of the NIH's National Heart, Lung, and Blood Institute, called the findings "very good news" for the roughly 2,500 children—and their families—with sickle cell who may be at risk of stroke.

### b. Increased hematocrit
**Type of risk factor:** Nonpreventable
**Strength of evidence:** Well established
**Treatment:** Possible
**Importance:** Limited

*Hematocrit* is a medical term for "red blood cell count." Under a microscope, blood isn't at all the way it looks to the naked eye. The liquid portion—plasma—is the color of straw. Suspended in plasma are white blood cells, which help the body fight infection, and red blood cells, which carry oxygen throughout the body. Most people's blood is about 45 to 50 percent red blood cells, but the normal level typically ranges from as low as 37 percent in some females to as high as 52 percent in some males. Regardless of gender, persons in the upper ranges have a higher-than-average risk of stroke because having that many red blood cells makes the blood thicker and thus more prone to clog blood vessels. Medical treatment exists for increased hematocrit, but its effectiveness is questionable.

### c. High fibrinogen
**Type of risk factor:** Nonpreventable
**Strength of evidence:** Suggestive
**Treatment:** Limited
**Importance:** Limited

When a teenager nicks himself the first time he shaves, it may be embarrassing. But thanks to fibrinogen, it's usually not life-threatening. Fibrinogen is a protein that helps blood clot. When we cut ourselves, fibrinogen turns into long fibrous strands that mesh together to form a clot. The clot plugs a bleeding blood vessel like a miniature Band-Aid. Understandably, persons with high fibrinogen levels can be prone to strokes because their blood clots too easily.

### d. High hemoglobin
**Type of risk factor:** Nonpreventable
**Strength of evidence:** Well established
**Treatment:** Limited
**Importance:** Limited

When television commercials use the phrase "iron-poor blood," they are really referring to hemoglobin. Hemoglobin is an iron-containing pigment found in red blood cells. In fact, hemoglobin is what gives red blood cells their bright red color. Some people's blood happens to be high in hemoglobin, which literally weighs down the red blood cells just enough to make the blood thicker than normal. Like blood with too many red cells, high-hemoglobin blood circulates sluggishly and tends to block blood vessels.

### e. Bloodstream fats
**Type of risk factor:** Preventable and nonpreventable aspects
**Strength of evidence:** Suggestive
**Treatment:** Value not established
**Importance:** Limited

Fatty deposits in the arteries are the major cause of ischemic stroke. So you might expect that people whose blood is rich in fats such as cholesterol and triglycerides are prone to stroke. Oddly, though, researchers have found no direct association between the two, except perhaps for men under the age of fifty. High levels of bloodstream fats are clearly potent risk factors for heart disease and atherosclerosis, however, which in turn are risk factors for stroke.

Once you understand that too many bloodstream fats can increase your risk of stroke, you'll understand why prescription medicines that lower cholesterol also lower your risk of stroke. Doctor prescribe drugs like Zocor and Pravachol, which reduce the amount of "bad" cholesterol in your system, to prevent heart attacks. But the medicines also reduce the incidence of stroke by about 27 percent, say researchers, by cleaning and protecting your arteries.

### 14. Oral contraceptives
**Type of risk factor:** Preventable
**Strength of evidence:** Suggestive
**Treatment:** Value not established
**Importance:** Limited

Sometimes two competent researchers can examine the same information but emerge with very different conclusions. In the 1960s, scientists noticed increasing numbers of stroke patients who had used oral contraceptives. By the 1970s and early 1980s, several studies had confirmed that taking birth control pills did indeed increase a woman's risk for later stroke by anywhere from four to thirteen times. But when Dr. Diana Pettiti of the Centers for Disease Control examined the evidence, she realized that many of the stroke patients were also cigarette smokers, which made her wonder whether the increased stroke risk came from the contraceptives or the smoking. Likewise, other investigators found no increase in women's stroke rates since the 1960s, when oral contraceptives became generally available in the United States. When an American Heart Association subcommittee on stroke examined risk factors in 1984, oral contraceptives emerged as the most controversial topic. In the end, the committee deadlocked.

### 15. Poverty
**Type of risk factor:** Frequently nonpreventable
**Strength of evidence:** Suggestive
**Treatment:** Value not established
**Importance:** Limited

African-Americans are disproportionately poor; 30 percent of blacks live below the poverty line compared to 10 percent of whites. And we also suffer more than our share of strokes. It's tempting to conclude that poverty and stroke are related. After all, if you're black and poor, you stand a greater chance of dying from a stroke than if you're black and affluent.

As international health expert Dr. Vicente Navarro of Johns Hopkins University reminds us, "How people live, get sick, and die depends not only on their race, sex, and age, but also on the class to which they belong."

But the evidence on stroke and poverty is mixed. One Baltimore study showed that affluent black males actually faced a *higher* risk of stroke than did poor white males, which suggests that wealth alone isn't enough to overcome other risk factors that hurt black men. In Great Britain as well, rich people get *more* strokes than do poor people.

If poverty is a risk factor for stroke, it may be indirect. When residents of Evans County, Georgia, were surveyed to measure how bothered they were by low energy, pounding heartbeat, "all kinds of ailments in different parts of your body," and other signs of distress, blacks tended to have higher scores than whites, and females higher scores than males. This may point to a higher level of stress-related and other disorders—including risk factors for stroke—that are caused by poverty.

### 16. Geographic location
**Type of risk factor:** Often nonpreventable
**Strength of evidence:** Suggestive
**Treatment:** Not feasible
**Importance:** Limited

People have strokes throughout the country. But your risk of stroke depends in some measure on where you live. In the swampy flats of Florida, the stroke rate is about the same as throughout the country as a whole. But step across the border into neighboring Georgia, and the rate is among the highest in the country. In fact, stroke is so prevalent in the Southeast that in 1990, alarmed federal and state investigators designated ten southeastern states, plus Oklahoma and Indiana, the "Stroke Belt" (Figure 11). Here, blacks are twice as likely as whites—and more likely than blacks living elsewhere—to die of stroke.

Investigators don't understand all the reasons why stroke is particularly prevalent in the Stroke Belt, but they have a few clues. For one, black women in the region have more hypertension than do black women elsewhere, and they do not control their high blood pressure as well. Another reason is that both black men and women are far heavier in the Southeast: the rates of obesity for black men and women with hypertension are 36 percent and 58 percent nationally; in the Southeast, the corresponding rates are 45 percent and 71 percent. The more you weigh, the more medicine it takes to control high blood pressure. And that means black people who are overweight suffer more side effects from antihypertension medicines—side effects that discourage them from taking the medicine as prescribed. Hypertension and obesity, of course, are risk factors for stroke.

The high stroke rate might also be tied to diet, because Southern blacks who move north continue to have more high blood pressure and obesity than do Northern-born blacks. Southern cooking may be delicious, but the sad fact is that much of it isn't the best for our health. Sausage and hot buttered grits, greens simmered with ham hocks, crisp fried chicken—they're all loaded with saturated fat, cholesterol, and sodium that our bodies don't need. Too often, the end result is hypertension, obesity, and eventually stroke.

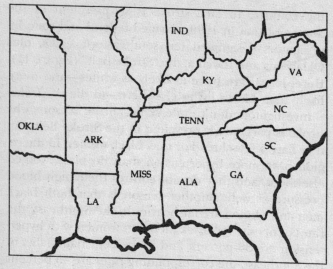

Figure 11. The Stroke Belt

The death rate from stroke is relatively low in New England, the northern Midwest, and the Mountain states.

## 17. Season and climate
**Type of risk factor:** Nonpreventable
**Strength of evidence:** Suggestive
**Treatment:** Value not established
**Importance:** Limited

Believe it or not, the weather appears to influence stroke rates. When the weather is pleasant, not many people die of stroke. But after a heat wave, and particularly during the winter months, doctors know to expect stroke patients. Japan has the highest rate of stroke deaths in the world, but Japanese people living in Hawaii's moderate climate have lower death rates from stroke.

Why temperature extremes bring on strokes is a medical mystery. But one educated guess is that temperatures in the sixties and seventies are the ideal working range for the cardiovascular system. When the mercury drops much below or above this comfort zone, the heart and blood vessels do not function as efficiently. This may be a reason why your blood pressure increases during the winter months. Uncontrolled hypertension, of course, is a risk factor for stroke.

18. **Physical inactivity**
     **Type of risk factor:** Preventable
     **Strength of evidence:** Suggestive
     **Treatment:** Value not established
     **Importance:** Limited

The evidence tying stroke to a sedentary lifestyle is inconsistent. Some research shows no link. Yet the Framingham Heart Study found a slight increase in stroke risk for inactive people. Elsewhere in New England, the same landmark study of former college students that named smoking as a risk factor in stroke also discovered that stroke patients were less likely to have participated in varsity sports as undergraduates. Physical activity is one of the least studied of all risk factors for stroke.

## COMBINATIONS OF RISK FACTORS

So when it comes to stroke, there are lots of risk factors to think about. What do they all mean? Consider this: If you are driving a car with broken turn signals, there is a chance that you will be stopped by the police.

### Is Heat Stroke a Stroke?

Heat stroke and stroke have two things in common: they are serious medical emergencies and they strike suddenly. (That's why they're called "stroke.") Other than that, heat stroke and stroke are two very different animals. Heat stroke occurs when the body becomes so overheated that it loses its ability to cool itself by evaporating sweat. Often patients will have spent long stretches in the hot sun without properly acclimating themselves to the heat. Heat stroke also occurs in humid weather, when sweat cannot easily evaporate. Heat stroke can cause a person's body temperature to rise to 107° F, a temperature that can cause fatal brain damage if not treated immediately by stripping the patient of their clothes, wrapping them in a water-soaked sheet and fanning them to cool them down, and summoning emergency care. There are lots of ways to prevent a stroke, but only one way to prevent heat stroke: acclimate gradually to the weather.

On the other hand, if your car has no turn signals, no headlights, no brakes, and no doors, your chances of a run-in with the law are greatly increased. Risks add up; every additional risk that you take places you in further jeopardy of being arrested.

So it is with stroke (and other diseases). When a doctor examines a patient, she may find a single risk factor for stroke—hypertension, say, or a family history of stroke. But more often, she'll find multiple risk factors, particularly in older persons. A male diabetic will be fearful because his mother died of stroke (three risk factors), or an elderly smoker with hypertension will complain of chest pain that indicates a chronic heart condition (four risk factors). These risk factors are additive; the more a person has, the more likely he or she is of suffering a stroke—and the more important it is to work aggressively to minimize the risk factors that can be controlled.

Doctors know that certain combinations of risk factors are particularly dangerous. "There is evidence that some [risk factors] become more important when in combination," says Dr. Mark L. Dyken, "and some are only important when in combination with others." In the late 1960s, researchers reported that while high blood pressure was the most important risk factor for stroke, the three-way combination of hypertension, smoking, and a certain weight distribution increased a person's chances of the disease by a factor of eight. Experts on oral contraceptives say that for women over thirty-five years of age, smoking cigarettes and taking birth control pills is a particularly volatile combination.

Later in this chapter, we'll review how one of the latest studies on multiple risk factors can help you estimate your chances of suffering a stroke. But first, let's see how multiple risk factors explain why stroke is so prevalent in the black community.

## AFRICAN-AMERICANS AT RISK

Modern-day tragedies such as the AIDS epidemic and the rise in unwanted early pregnancies can obscure the fact that medicine has scored some startling successes in the past twenty years. The war on stroke is clearly one of them. The incidence of stroke has declined bit by bit since the turn of the century, and particularly since around 1970, thanks to better antihypertensive therapy, a decline in heart disease, more people who've quit smoking, and greater public awareness of stroke. In fact, from 1973 to 1981 alone, six hundred thousand Americans—enough to fill a good-sized city—who would have had strokes if the rate hadn't declined, were spared the disease. And in the past fifteen years, stroke deaths in the United States population as a whole have been cut in half.

Much of the improvement has benefited people of color. In fact, the stroke rate has plummeted in the African-American community (particularly for women) faster than among whites. But black people are still at greater risk. "Blacks still succumb to stroke three to six times more often than whites," reminds Dr. Charles K. Francis of Harlem Hospital Medical Center "[And] strokes occur in blacks at an earlier age." While 11 percent of deaths among white Americans are from stroke, 13 percent of blacks deaths are caused by stroke. Death rates from hemorrhage, thrombosis, and embolism—the major types of stroke—are all higher in blacks than in whites.

One of the more illuminating insights on race and stroke emerged from a 1989 study in Allegheny County, Pennsylvania, where Pittsburgh is located. Investigators from the University of Pittsburgh teamed up with colleagues from Meharry Medical College in Nashville, Tennessee, to study the factors that best predict how many cases of stroke will occur in a given geographic area. The researchers knew that socioeconomic status is a risk factor for stroke, so they analyzed data for such items as family income, education, and unemployment. In the end, what was the best predictor of stroke rates in a given area? The percentage of black residents.

Does Africa provide any clues about why stroke is so common among African-Americans? There, too, stroke is prevalent among blacks, although this may not have always been the case. As early as 1929, doctors reported a startlingly low incidence of hypertension in Africans. "These early observations soon became the exception rather than the rule," says Dr. O.O. Akinkugbe of the Department of Medicine at the University of Ibadan in Nigeria. "In most parts of Africa in the last three decades, the prevalence of high [blood] pressure does not differ in important respects from that in black and white communities elsewhere in the world." The overall incidence of stroke seems to be increasing as well, although accurate information on African disease rates is difficult to come by. These increases in stroke and hypertension may be linked to the many changes brought by urbanization: more atherosclerosis, different diet, more consumption of salt and alcohol, less exercise, and so forth.

But even among contemporary Africans, the risk of stroke is no match for that of African-Americans. In fact, although Americans as a whole have one of the lowest stroke death rates of any industrialized country, black Americans have one of the highest stroke rates in the world.

That one statistic tells you a lot about how devastating life in America can be for black people. African-Americans carry many of the same strong genes as Africans, but too many of us die too young. Racism and bias against the poor show in a hundred different stressful ways—bad schools, inadequate police protection, limited access to loans for better housing and college educations, and certainly inferior health care. On top of that, we're sometimes our own worst enemy, because we don't treat our bodies with respect. We smoke too much, drink too much, and eat too much of the wrong kind of food. Instead of trying to prevent illness, we delay seeing a doctor until a disease is in an advanced stage and we simply can't stand the pain any longer. And the closest we get to exercise is watching it on TV.

Life for African-Americans adds up to one thing— risk factors, and lots of them. That's why we get sick and die before our time. Take hypertension, for example. High blood pressure, the most important treatable risk factor for stroke, is rampant in the black community. "Hypertension *is* different in black people," stressed the editor of the *Journal of the American Medical Association* in an editorial over twenty years ago. "It develops earlier in life, is frequently more severe, and results in a higher mortality at a younger age, more commonly from strokes than from coronary artery disease."

Compared to whites, blacks also have more heart disease and sickle cell anemia. Black people drink more excessively and smoke cigarettes more often, although whites smoke more cigarettes in total. Obesity is more common in African-Americans, particularly women. Researchers also tell us that black people have a higher incidence of disease of certain arteries inside the brain. All of these factors place blacks at significantly higher risk of a stroke.

The prevalence of risk factors in the black community may also point to the failure of efforts to educate all Americans about stroke and how to avoid it. With hypertension, for example, a national education campaign launched in 1973 by the U.S. Department of Health and Human Services is credited with much of the decrease in hypertension and hypertension-related diseases (such as stroke) over the past two decades. But deaths from the complications of hypertension are still six to thirteen times greater in blacks than in whites.

## MORE STROKES THAN WE THOUGHT

In 1998, scientists who studied one year's worth of health records for Cleveland, Ohio, announced that more strokes occur every year in America than previously believed. By examining a city whose black population is typical of the rest of the nation, the researchers suggested that the national estimate of 500,000 strokes per year, which is based on the Framingham Heart Study, should be revised upward to 700,000 strokes. The reasons for the higher stroke figures? Experts blame the higher blood pressure in the African-American community; more smoking, obesity, and poverty; and possibly genetic differences in African-Americans compared to whites.

Dr. Charles K. Francis of the Harlem Hospital Medical Center believes this lingering disparity remains partly because of the apparent failure of national health education programs to reach and teach blacks and Hispanics. "As a result, more whites than blacks are aware of their hypertension, are receiving treatment, and are well controlled," suggests Dr. Francis.

The lack of information shows up in health surveys. When pollster Lou Harris asked people to name the major causes of heart disease, he found that blacks and whites alike knew that hypertension, stress, and too much alcohol led to heart trouble. But blacks were less likely to identify obesity, cigarette smoking, lack of exercise, and too much cholesterol. Similarly, blacks and Hispanics know less about nutrition and are less concerned about their eating habits, according to annual telephone surveys by *Prevention* magazine. And according to the U.S. Department of Health and Human Services, African-Americans are less likely than whites to know what a normal blood-pressure reading is, which may be because doctors tend to describe black patients' blood pressure to them in general terms ("high," "borderline," "normal") rather than use actual numbers.

Nevertheless, once we have accurate information, there is a great deal that we can do to minimize the risk factors that may be stacked against us. Take a look at this summary of risk factors discussed in this chapter:

## Risk Factors for Stroke

A. Well-established risk factors
   1. Treatable or at least partly preventable
      a. Hypertension
      b. Heart disease
      c. Prior stroke
      d. Increased hematocrit
      e. Sickle cell anemia
      f. Alcohol consumption
      g. Diabetes
      h. Cigarette smoking
      i. Obesity
      j. Cocaine
   2. Nonpreventable or treatment value not established
      a. Age
      b. Gender
      c. Stroke in family
      d. High hemoglobin
      e. Asymptomatic bruit
B. Suggestive evidence
   1. Treatable or at least partly preventable
      a. Serum lipids
      b. Oral contraceptives
      c. Poverty
      d. Physical inactivity
   2. Nonpreventable or treatment value not established
      a. Geographic location

b. Season and climate
c. High fibrinogen

Of twenty-two risk factors, fourteen are treatable or at least partly preventable. Even more important, nine of the most important risk factors are treatable or preventable, and that means that blacks at risk of stroke can do a great deal to protect themselves. There are treatment centers and self-help programs for persons

---

### If You Have a Migraine, Are You Headed for a Stroke?

Few burdens cause as much misery as a migraine headache. A typical attack can mean hours or even days of irritability, nausea and vomiting, and above all, searing pain. Some migraine sufferers may be in such distress that they fear they are on the verge of a stroke. After all, one of the reasons people get headaches is that blood vessels inside their head expand and press on sensitive nerve tissue—the same basic mechanism behind some strokes.

Then are migraines and strokes related? For most people, the answer, thankfully, is no. When Drs. Thomas Tatemichi and J.P. Mohr of the New York Neurological Institute combed the medical literature, they found that 96 percent of the ischemic strokes in young adults had nothing to do with migraines. The researchers didn't survey elderly patients or persons with cerebral hemorrhages, but it's probably safe to assume that for these patients, too, migraines don't cause strokes.

The tricky thing about migraines is that they can cause stroke-like symptoms. Migraines can cause visual disturbances, abnormal limb sensations, weakness and numbness in one half of a person's body, and a host of other problems characteristic of strokes. To complicate the picture, some bona fide strokes are indeed accompanied by severe headache.

Anyone who has a problem with migraines would do well to consult a physician, preferably a specialist in internal medicine or neurology. These doctors are trained to distinguish migraines from strokes. If a migraine is just a migraine (and the vast majority of them are), a doctor can help treat the pain—and usually give the patient peace of mind.

addicted to nicotine, alcohol, or cocaine. Hospitals and community health centers often offer free screening for hypertension and sickle cell anemia. Regular consultation with a physician or other health professional can prevent, detect, and treat heart disease and diabetes. Appendix B explains how you can get additional help.

We've come a long way since Hippocrates wrote this description of what was probably a subarachnoid hemorrhage:

> When persons in good health are suddenly seized with pains in the head, and straightaway are laid down speechless . . . they die in seven days . . .

True, stroke still takes a terrible toll in human life and suffering—a burden disproportionately felt in the black community. And granted, we can't completely control our risk of having a stroke (or any other disease, for that matter). But we do know a great deal more about stroke today than we have in years past, and one of the lessons is that when it comes to beating the odds, a great deal of the power lies in our own hands. Even if we or people we love have a stroke, there's a lot that doctors can do to help patients recover. And there's a lot that we can do to help ourselves. In the next chapter, we'll discuss what to do when someone has a stroke.

# CHAPTER 3

# When Stroke Strikes

In August 1987, Phillip Mason, Ph.D., an African-American artist, was heading to work on the first day of his new job as academic dean of the Art Institute of Southern California. His excitement over his new position would soon turn to bewilderment. "I had just left my office with two of my paintings," remembers the artist, "when suddenly, and without warning, I felt a sickening wave of dizziness." Mason collapsed to the floor, his efforts to regain the use of his feet reduced to slow-motion frustration. His wife phoned for help, and paramedics quickly arrived and hooked him to life support. "There was a period of haziness," Mason would later write in the National Stroke Association's newsletter *Be Stroke Smart*. "And all I remember was the ride in the ambulance with the siren screaming."

After months of hard work, Mason recovered completely from a stroke that had paralyzed half of his body, left him with a whisper of a voice, and riddled his memory so severely that he couldn't remember where he had gotten his Ph.D. It was a long and difficult road, one filled with frustration and achievement, despair over the agony of physical therapy ("physical torture," as Mason called it), and delight over small triumphs like learning to tie his shoes again.

It's often said that a long journey begins with a single step. For Phillip Mason, that step was getting immediate medical care. He didn't wait to see if the mysterious symptoms might go away. He didn't discourage his wife from making a fuss over him. He allowed himself to be taken to a doctor right away.

Thousands of people have strokes each day. For many, the event comes with no warning, no signal of the fate that lies in store. Even when there are the tell-tale warning signs of a transient ischemic attack (TIA), many fail to understand that this temporary condition is often a prelude to a more massive stroke. "Every day I see patients who had warning signs but didn't recognize them," Dr. James Toole of the Bowman Gray School of Medicine in Winston-Salem, North Carolina, told *Newsweek*.

According to a Gallup poll, 97 percent of Americans don't know the warning signs of stroke. Because they miss the significance of what they are experiencing, many stroke patients—especially those who have had a TIA, which is fleeting and causes no permanent brain damage—delay seeking medical care or fail to seek it altogether. They may assume that the reason behind the brief sensation of numbness or muscle weakness is trivial. They tell themselves they're working too hard, skipping breakfast too often, staying up too late at night. Regrettably, over half of all stroke patients fail to go to a hospital within twenty-four hours of the stroke, according to the National Stroke Association.

But laypersons aren't the only ones who overlook strokes. Doctors make errors, too. A 1988 study of 182 deaths at hospitals owned by American Medical International of Beverly Hills, California, found that nine people died simply because their strokes were diagnosed as something else. The reverse is true as well: sometimes other illnesses masquerade as a stroke. Even at Toronto's MacLachan Acute Stroke Unit, one of the few specialized intensive-care facilities for stroke in North America, researchers admit that the rate of misdiagnosis is substantial. "About 15 percent of patients admitted do not have stroke," say Drs. J.G. D'Alton and J.W. Norris of the University of Ottowa and the University of Toronto, respectively. What the patients actually have typically ranges from unrecognized seizures and mental confusion to fainting or a sudden loss of strength—none of it stroke-related. Hypoglycemia (low blood sugar) causes drowsiness and sometimes coma, which is sometimes mistaken for the impaired consciousness of a stroke. Tumors can press on certain regions of the brain and mimic the impaired brain function of a stroke. Sometimes epileptic fits cause paralysis on one side of the body—an obvious similarity with stroke.

The best way for a doctor to avoid misdiagnosing a stroke is to take a patient's history thoroughly and carefully. This way, the doctor learns the nature of any risk factors, which reveal much about a patient's likelihood for stroke. At many hospitals and other health care facilities, strokes are diagnosed with little error. Unfortunately, public hospitals—the only facilities that will treat many inner-city people of color and the poor—are typically so understaffed, underfunded, and overcrowded that the quality of care suffers.

"The poor must use [medical] institutions . . . that are certainly not designed to make it easy for anyone,

## What to Do When Someone Has a Stroke

These are the classic signs of stroke:

- Deterioration in vision, speech, comprehension, or sensation, lasting seconds to hours.
- Sudden weakness, loss of sensation, or complete paralysis in one limb or in an arm and a leg, with or without involvement of the face.
- Sudden blurred vision (especially if only in one eye), slurred speech, unexplained dizziness, incoordination, sudden falls, difficulty swallowing, vomiting.
- Headache that accompanies the above symptoms.
- Sudden loss of consciousness (not caused by an injury).

If you or someone you know shows these signs, get medical help immediately, no matter how minor the symptoms or how briefly they last.

Why is immediate care so important? One of the reasons is that brain tissue can survive longer without oxygen than researchers have historically believed. The traditional thinking was that neurons begin to die if they are deprived of oxygen for more than a few minutes. Recent research suggests that this "five-minute rule" is no longer valid. Paramedics have been able to save stroke patients whose brains have been deprived of oxygen for as long as ninety minutes. This means that doctors have more time to intervene before brain damage becomes irreversible. So the sooner a patient gets to a doctor, the greater the chances that lasting damage can be prevented.

While an ambulance is on the way, help the person lie down. In severe strokes, the patient may have difficulty breathing, so watch the person carefully. They may need cardiopulmonary resuscitation (CPR); if you are not familiar with this simple lifesaving procedure, find someone who is. Elevating the head and shoulders with a pillow or folded blanket can ease minor breathing problems.

Stroke patients sometimes feel nauseous and vomit. If this happens, turn their head to one side and help clear their mouths to guard against their inhaling vomited material—a potential cause of pneumonia. It's a good idea not to let the patient eat or drink anything.

Paralysis may leave the stroke patient with no control over the arms and legs, so protect paralyzed limbs from harm.

A prayer may help with events to come.

(Adapted from *The Mayo Clinic Family Health Book*. William Morrow, 1990, New York City. David E. Larson, Editor.)

much less the poorly educated, socially disorganized patient," writes Dr. Margaret Heagerty of Harlem Hospital in the *Journal of Health Care for the Poor and Underserved*. "All of us in the trenches of medical care for the poor can tell war stories about institutional ineptitude and callousness: block appointments, long waiting times at clinics, lack of interpreters for Spanish patients, and perhaps the most serious, an attitude that is more than a little authoritarian, . . . a mixture of colonialism and punitiveness."

Many facilities clearly do a heroic job with the resources they have, and not all staffs are insensitive. But the fact remains that blacks are much less likely than others to have access to high-quality care, including care from neurologists who specialize in stroke. Studies show that the elapsed time from the onset of stroke symptoms to arrival in a hospital is longer for persons of color than for whites. Indeed, black people who suffer strokes are often not hospitalized at all, and when we are, we frequently receive second-class treatment. Dr. Edgar Kenton of Philadelphia's Lankenau Hospital stresses that many minority senior citizens could afford a private physician if their Medicare payments were bolstered with supplementary health insurance. "But often they are admitted from emergency rooms to the teaching services as unassigned patients to be followed thereafter by residents in the outpatient clinics and not as private patients," says Dr. Kenton. "Thus, they have limited access to more experienced physicians."

Limited access to good care may have been one reason that a 1987 study found that for Medicare patients, the death rates from stroke at fifteen Southern California hospitals ranged from 23.6 percent to

## Making the System Work for You

If you're black or poor or both, you may find that the health care system isn't providing for your needs. But that doesn't mean you can't improve your chances of getting good care. Dr. Charles K. Francis of the Harlem Hospital Medical Center offers this advice to patients:

1. Be sure to ask the doctor what's wrong.

Some doctors don't communicate well with patients. They may assume that the less the patient knows, the better. Or they may doubt the patient's ability to understand certain information. A patient may wait for hours to see a doctor, then sit through an examination and tests, only to be told, "It's not serious." If that happens to you, ask what the problem *is*. If the doctor is still vague, ask for specific information. ("What was my blood pressure?" "Am I having a stroke?" "Will I feel better?")

2. Ask for the evidence for and against.

To evaluate a patient, doctors weigh all sorts of information. They consider the person's history, their present health, any risk factors for certain diseases, and the results of tests. Often information is suggestive but not definitive; sometimes one piece of information even contradicts another. The diagnosis a doctor reaches is often less than 100 percent certain. It's good to know how strongly the evidence points one way or the other. If there's a fair amount of uncertainty, you may want to get a second opinion.

3. Ask specific questions about what you should do next.

Sometimes patients are sent home without being told what they should do to follow up on a problem. Often their condition worsens. Ask your doctor what you should do to regain your health. Don't be afraid to ask for very specific instructions ("Should I do anything after I leave your office?" "Are there things I can do at home to help myself feel better?" "When I make another appointment, should I come back here? Which doctor should I see?") The more you know, the better you will be able to help yourself.

34.8 percent—much higher than the 15.6 percent statewide average, according to San Francisco–based California Medical Review, Inc. The hospitals replied that many Medicare patients are sicker than others, so you'd expect a higher death rate. But even the California Association of Hospitals and Health Systems, a trade group for the industry, admitted that the findings might pinpoint problems in how hospitals treat elderly, low-income Medicare patients.

Given these handicaps, what can black stroke patients and their families do to ensure that a stroke is diagnosed accurately? For any medical problem, one of the most important ways to help ensure a high quality of care is to interact with the medical staff. If you have information that may be relevant to the patient's condition, volunteer it. If you don't understand why a procedure is being performed, ask. If the explanation still doesn't make sense to you, don't hesitate to ask again. It's easy to feel intimidated in a hospital, a place with unfamiliar procedures and mystifying language. This is particularly true for many people of color and the poor, who may feel particularly unempowered and reluctant to speak up. But the people who get the most out of medical care are the ones who become active participants in the process.

Likewise, it's important to be attentive while the patient is receiving care. A stroke is often a considerably difficult medical emergency for friends and family as well as for the patient. Given the suddenness of many strokes and the frequently devastating health effects, it is natural to be deeply concerned over the well-being of a loved one. But it is also important to stay alert. Hospital care is a human endeavor, and mistakes can happen even in the best of institutions. Knowing how the medical staff should handle stroke cases can help you evaluate whether the patient is receiving good care. That's what this chapter is all about.

## ENTERING THE HOSPITAL

Anyone who has had a stroke should be admitted to a hospital, even if the stroke was a TIA and even if they feel fine afterward. Medical care should begin as soon as the patient comes through the door, and even sooner if the patient was transported by an ambulance. If the numbness, nausea, or other symptoms worsen, the medical team knows that the stroke is still "in progress." Their goal in this case is to keep the patient alive and comfortable and to do what they can to prevent any brain damage from becoming more extensive. If the patient is having trouble breathing, doctors may insert a tube in the throat to help maintain an airway. If hypertension is contributing to a hemorrhage, they may administer medicine to control it. Certain fluids may be given intravenously, and the medical staff may insert a catheter (a long flexible tube) into the urethra to help a patient who has difficulty with bladder control. Many stroke patients develop what doctors call *contractures*, in which the muscles in a patient's hand, foot, or other body part flex in a rigid spasm. The medical staff can help manage these.

For years, doctors took their time when examining stroke patients. There was little a medical team could do to prevent a stroke from worsening, so there was no reason to rush. Nowadays, new medicines and therapies for recent stroke patients mean that speed is of the essence. Once brain tissue begins to lose its supply of oxygen and glucose, it starts to die. And if these nutrients are denied for too long, the tissue dies permanently. But if the medical team can restore the blood supply quickly enough, even nutrient-starved brain tissue can recover. Dr. Peritz Scheinberg of the University of Miami School of Medicine suggests that given the limits of medical science, the so-called "window of opportunity" is narrow indeed. "Present evidence indicates that, unless a way is found to initiate treatment within minutes or one to two hours, effective stroke treatment will elude us." Writing in the journal *Neurology,* Dr. Scheinberg notes that one hospital (University of Cincinnati) managed to reduce the amount of time it takes to evaluate patients and begin all-important drug therapy from nearly ten hours to just fifty-four minutes—a time savings of 90 percent. As other hospitals follow suit, and as researchers develop better treatments, more and more patients will reap the benefits of such streamlined care. (Chapter 6 discusses some of the new experimental treatments for stroke.)

At some point, a physician takes a detailed history of the patient. There may not be time for this during the so-called "acute" stages of the disease, when everyone is busy tending to the patient's immediate and urgent needs. But a physician should return when the patient is more stable (in which case the stroke is referred to as "completed") and ask the patient (or a family member) a series of questions about the patient's risk factors, immediate and former symptoms, and lifestyle. (See page 89.) The answers to these questions help establish a foundation for deciding how to best manage the patient's care and recuperation. In any given case, physicians may feel that, based on their experience and judgment, they can accurately diagnose and begin to care for a stroke patient without asking each one of these questions. It may also be acceptable—and even preferable—to ask the questions over a period of time instead of during a single session. The questions are listed here to help a patient and family members appreciate the approach that a physician should use to assess the patient's condition and determine its cause. One of the best ways to help the doctor is to describe the symptoms as specifically and carefully as possible.

Stroke patients routinely receive a physical exam to check vital signs (blood pressure in both arms, temperature, and breathing); the status of the lungs, skin, and heart; and the presence of any pain. A physician gently touches the neck, jaw, and head, feeling for an abnormal pulse in the carotid and temporal arteries that could be a sign of obstruction. The eyes may be examined. Doctors make an extensive check of the nerves, especially the nerves of the head. This involves testing various parts of the body for strength, reflexes, and range of motion. Doctors check the patient's mental state and listen for speech problems. They note whether the patient has bladder and bowel control.

Doctors typically order a number of routine laboratory tests, and patients will have to give blood and urine samples. Blood tests measure how well the blood clots and whether the number of red blood cells falls within a normal range. A portion of the blood goes to measure the presence of heart enzymes, which can be a warning sign for heart damage. A portion is also used to test for venereal disease, since stroke can be an early sign of syphilis. A urine test measures the presence of glucose, proteins, blood, and other substances in the urine, which can give a doctor clues about such possible disorders as glucose

## Questions Doctors Should Ask
## Stroke Patients or Their Families

Questions about a patient's present state:

1. Does any part of your body feel weak? Numb? In pain? Otherwise abnormal?
2. Do you have difficulty talking? Reading? Writing?
3. Have you had seizures? Memory disturbances?
4. Are you having any visual problems?
5. Does the room seem to be spinning? Are you having trouble keeping your balance, or hearing?
6. Do you have a headache, nausea, or vomiting?

Questions about the stroke:

1. What were you doing when the stroke occurred?
2. Did the problems happen suddenly or gradually?
3. How long did the symptoms last? Did they get worse over time?
4. Have you ever experienced these problems before?
5. Have you lost consciousness? Had changes in mood or behavior? Changes in speech or other neurological problems?

Questions about the patient's background:

1. Do you or does your family have a history of:
   Hypertension?
   Heart disease?
   Diabetes?
   Thyroid disease?
   Atherosclerosis (hardening of the arteries)?
   Blood disorders, including sickle cell anemia?
   Seizures?
   Migraines?
   Besides the problems that brought you to the hospital today, do you have any other illnesses?
2. Do you smoke? Drink alcohol? How much and how often?
3. What medications and other drugs do you use? For women: Do you take birth control pills?
4. Are your financial arrangements secure? Have you suffered recent losses? Tell me about your family. What community activities are you engaged in? Tell me about your work, your hobbies, your leisure activities.

SOURCES: Adapted from Dunkle, R.E., Schmidley, J.W., eds., *Stroke in the Elderly*. Copyright © 1987 by Springer Publishing Company, Inc., New York 10012, used by permission, p. 75, and Meyer. J.S., Shaw, T., *Diagnosis and Management of Stroke and TIAs*. Addison Wesley, 1982, pp. 79–80.

intolerance, which is a possible sign of diabetes—a risk factor in stroke.

If they have the equipment, doctors use sophisticated technology to diagnose strokes. CT scans, MR images, and a number of other tests and procedures are invaluable tools that help physicians determine whether a person has suffered a stroke and, if so, the location and extent of the damage. Fifteen years ago, it wasn't uncommon for strokes to be misdiagnosed. Cerebral hemorrhages were correctly diagnosed only 32 percent of the time (and ischemias 88 percent of the time) during bedside observation, according to one study of 206 consecutive stroke patients. Today, this new technology allows doctors to pinpoint strokes with much greater precision than ever before.

Naturally, any given test has its weak points and strong points. One procedure might be well suited to show whether a patient has a certain kind of stroke but not another kind. A second procedure might present a patient with certain risks but be able to deliver information quickly. These strengths and limitations of diagnostic tests are important, because blacks and whites typically have different kinds of stroke. Dr. Louis R. Caplan, a neurologist with the Tufts University School of Medicine in Boston, and a leader in the study of racial differences in stroke, says that while whites have more strokes from clogged neck arteries, blacks are more prone to strokes affecting the cerebral arteries, which surround and penetrate the brain. Strokes in cerebral arteries often come about as a result of diabetes and uncontrolled hypertension (both of which are more prevalent in the black community) and do not commonly cause TIAs (which are relatively rare among blacks). Another racial difference: blacks, particularly black men, have a higher incidence of hemorrhagic stroke because of the high prevalence of uncontrolled hypertension in the black community.

---

### Stroke and Syphilis

If you are old enough to remember the days before penicillin, you might recall the classic sign of syphilis: open skin sores. But many people don't realize that syphilis causes strokes, too. When the bacteria responsible for syphilis enter the body, they head for the blood vessels, which become inflamed and start to build scar tissue. If this scar tissue accumulates to the point of blocking an artery in the brain, the patient has a stroke.

A stroke is usually obvious. But the early stages of syphilis are not. So doctors like to check a stroke patient's blood for the telltale presence of antibodies—specialized infection-fighting cells mobilized by the body in response to a bacterial attack. If they find antibodies for the syphilis bacteria, they treat the stroke *and* the sexually transmitted disease.

Recent reports suggest that after a period of decline, syphilis cases are on the rise. Which may mean that doctors will begin to see more and more stroke patients whose medical problems are more than meets the eye.

---

Because the type and location of a stroke are partly governed by race, black and white patients often need different sorts of diagnostic tests. For example, invasive tests—those involving instruments that are inserted into the body—are good for detecting hardening and thickening of the arteries inside the head, while noninvasive tests are better for finding such atherosclerosis in the neck arteries and elsewhere. Since blacks typically have more cerebral artery disease, invasive tests are particularly well suited for black patients. "Noninvasive tests are relatively less useful in blacks and women," write Drs. Louis Caplan and Edward S. Cooper, "while angiography and CT are

even more important diagnostic tools in blacks."
Angiography involves injecting a dye into the arteries
so they will be visible on an X ray. Angiography is useful
for blacks because it shows the presence of lacunae and
other evidence of hypertension-related arterial disease
within the brain. CT scans are X rays of thin sections of
the body. CT scans are good because of their extraordinary capacity to detect hemorrhagic stroke, which is
more common in patients with hypertension.

## STARTING TREATMENT

The results of the diagnostic tests and laboratory
procedures will tell doctors whether the patient has
indeed suffered a stroke or whether the problem is
some other medical condition—like a seizure or what
doctors call a "confusional state"—that merely mimics
a stroke. These test results will also pinpoint whether a
stroke is a hemorrhage or an ischemia, and how
extensive the damage is. If the person has suffered a
TIA, the tests can help predict how imminent a more
massive stroke may be.

Once physicians understand what they are dealing
with, treatment begins in earnest. It's a lot harder to
treat a stroke than it is to prevent one. Strokes ignite a
chain of events in the brain that is difficult to interrupt (although researchers are developing promising
new ways to stop this deadly process, as we'll discuss in
Chapter 6).

So there's no magic pill a doctor can give a stroke
patient, no elixir to restore an ailing brain to health.
But by the same token, that doesn't mean doctors are
powerless, either. By keeping the patient as comfortable as possible, and addressing underlying medical

problems, doctors help position the patient for as complete a recovery as is possible.

You might think that doctors would naturally use different treatment strategies in black stroke patients. After all, stroke is different in blacks and whites. African-Americans tend to have more hemorrhagic strokes than do whites, and the strokes involve different blood vessels. Blacks have more strokes and die more often from them. Black stroke patients are more likely to have uncontrolled hypertension and to have a biochemical makeup that alters the effects of certain hypertension medicines.

Moreover, blacks are more likely to have serious health problems in addition to stroke—the immediate problem that brought them to a doctor's care. "Diabetes is more common in black stroke patients [than in white stroke patients]," says Dr. Edward S. Cooper of the Hospital of the University of Pennsylvania. "Hypertension is not only more common but also more severe." Heart disease, kidney disease, arthritis, peptic ulcer, and other illnesses are frequently found as well. All of these conditions make treating a stroke more difficult.

But researchers often fail to take these differences into account when devising strategies for treating stroke patients. "Most of the studies on stroke treatment have been conducted on whites," admits Dr. Louis Caplan of the Tufts University School of Medicine. "It was assumed that the findings applied to blacks as well."

What does this mean for the average black stroke patient? It means that while doctors may—and should—prescribe many of the same therapeutic measures for white and black stroke patients, black patients need an extra measure of consideration because of the effects of race. In the pages that follow, we'll hear more about how race can play an important factor in treating stroke. First, though, let's walk through the basics of what doctors try to do to help a stroke patient begin the road to recovery.

Doctors start by confining a stroke patient to bed. Strokes hurt the brain's ability to regulate the flow of blood to its tissues, and if a patient tries to stand soon after suffering a stroke, the normally slight drop in blood pressure can cause a significant drop in blood flow to the brain—thus worsening the stroke. Moreover, moving about raises a patient's blood pressure, and high blood pressure is a major cause of hemorrhagic strokes. In these patients, bed rest helps prevent continued or fresh bleeding.

## Treating TIAs

Transient ischemic attacks are rarer in blacks than they are in whites, but the treatment in either case is similar. TIAs caused by blood clots—the most common form of transient attack—can be attacked with so-called anticoagulant medicines or antiplatelet medicines, both of which help discourage the formation of clots. One of the more popular antiplatelet medicines today is common aspirin, which has properties of a blood thinner as well as a pain reliever. If the TIA is caused by debris that's partially blocking a carotid artery, doctors can remove the obstruction surgically. This operation is called a *carotid endarterectomy* [car-ah´-tid en-dar-ter-ect´-uh-mee]. ("Endarterium" is the thickened inside lining of a fat-clogged artery; "ectomy" means removal.) Surgeons can also bypass the obstruction by building an arterial bridge around it in a procedure similar to a heart bypass operation.

## Treating Other Ischemic Strokes

The goal behind treating ischemic stroke is to restore circulation to the areas of the brain that are cut off by a blood clot and to prevent further clots from forming. As in TIAs, anticoagulants can help, both by dissolving the blood clot that's causing the problem and by breaking up smaller blood clots that, if unattended, might eventually grow to obstruct an artery. Similarly, doctors may prescribe aspirin to help prevent specialized blood cells called platelets from sticking together and starting a clot. Doctors also use medicines called *vasodilators* ("vaso" refers to blood vessels; "dilate" means to open) to widen the arteries in the brain, which sometimes allows more blood to flow into damaged tissues via healthy blood vessels. Finally, as with TIAs, surgeons can perform a carotid endarterectomy to remove the fatty debris from a diseased artery, or they can build an alternate route around the obstruction.

## Treating Hemorrhagic Strokes

Cerebral hemorrhage—the type of stroke that blacks are particularly prone to—is also one of the most devastating. The death rate from this type of stroke is high, and many patients who survive the initial attack are severely disabled even before they reach a doctor's care. Once doctors determine that a person has suffered a hemorrhagic stroke, treatment can take several directions.

In most patients, controlling hypertension is all-important. Cerebral hemorrhage is usually caused by high blood pressure, so lowering the patient's blood pressure is key. When it comes to managing hypertension in blacks, some medicines are more effective than others. But medicine can control hypertension just as effectively in blacks as in whites, despite the fact that hypertension in blacks is often more severe. The trick is that many black patients have to work harder to be healthy. Black people are often more sensitive to sodium (salt) than are whites, which makes controlling hypertension more difficult. We often delay seeing a doctor until we are too sick to ignore a problem any longer, which means that an illness is more advanced—and harder to treat—by the time we seek care. The high cost of health care, the scarcity of physicians in black neighborhoods, difficulty in getting transportation to doctors' offices—these are all reasons why treating hypertension (and other health problems) in blacks can be a challenge.

For these reasons, doctors need to treat hypertension aggressively in black patients, and they need to understand what medicines work best. Dr. Elijah Saunders, a nationally recognized hypertension expert at the University of Maryland Hospital in Baltimore, recommends diuretics as first-line medicine for black hypertensive patients. These relatively inexpensive medicines lower blood pressure by reducing the amount of fluids in the bloodstream. As a second line of defense, medicines called beta blockers or ACE inhibitors are helpful, particularly when used in conjunction with diuretics. For stroke patients, the goal is to lower blood pressure aggressively but gradually. Reducing blood pressure too rapidly can cause problems.

In the meantime, patients are typically given medicine to help blood clot and to prevent further bleeding into the brain. Patients with headaches and restlessness—which are often severe with hemorrhagic strokes—may receive medicine to relieve pain and help them sleep.

Sometimes doctors use medicines or surgery to relieve the pressure that leaking blood places on nearby brain tissues. In fact, stroke expert Dr. Edward S. Cooper says that blacks who have hemorrhagic strokes usually need surgery for their condition to improve. For patients who have an aneurism that has not yet burst, surgeons can take a number of preventive measures, including tying off the arteries that feed it.

## CARING FOR THE WHOLE BODY

While the understandable focus of concern in stroke is the blood vessels leading into the brain, the rest of the body needs attention as well. Otherwise, life-threatening complications can set in. When patients die within a few weeks of suffering a stroke, the cause of death isn't always the stroke itself. Pneumonia, blood clots, and even urinary tract infections are often contributing factors. These conditions are preventable and treatable if they are caught early, and family members should ask the medical staff how they can help.

Many of these complications arise because the human body was designed to *move*. Immobility hurts the muscles, the bones, and every other body system. For example, healthy lung tissue contains a certain amount of fluid that usually circulates throughout the lung as a result of the motion of normal daily activities. When people are confined to bed, gravity causes this fluid to settle to the bottom of the lungs, where it can become a breeding ground for the viruses and bacteria that cause pneumonia. Likewise, patients who are comatose and unable to cough cannot remove excess fluid from their lungs. Stroke patients should be turned periodically so they don't lie on their back and on either side for more than two hours at a time. This helps prevent lung fluids from settling. Antibiotics can ensure that pneumonia is halted before it presents a threat. Another cause of pneumonia—inhaled food particles—is a potential danger in stroke patients who cannot swallow well or who have vomited. These patients can be fed through the nose with a *nasogastric* (commonly called "NG") *tube* or through a needle inserted directly into the bloodstream.

Immobility frequently causes blood clots to form in the deep veins of a paralyzed leg. Lack of activity makes blood circulation sluggish to begin with, because as we work our bodies during everyday activities such as walking, bending, and lifting, the rhythmic contraction of muscle tissue helps push blood through the arteries. In a paralyzed leg, circulation slows even more, hastening the development of clots. These can be fatal if they lodge in the artery that feeds blood to the lungs, a condition known as *pulmonary embolism*. Smaller clots can even lodge in the brain and cause a second stroke. Family members can help by preventing these clots from forming. Move the patient's legs periodically. If the hospital doesn't provide elastic stockings, buy some for the patient at a pharmacy. And make sure the patient drinks plenty of fluids, which helps by preventing the blood from getting too thick. Be sure to check with the medical staff before intervening with these or other measures.

Because stroke patients can lose the sensation of a full bladder or lose control over the muscles that prevent the bladder from emptying, medical personnel may insert a catheter into the urethra (the channel that carries urine from the bladder to the outside of the body). Sometimes these so-called "indwelling catheters" allow bacteria to enter the urinary tract, causing potentially serious urinary tract infections. Minimizing the amount of time that these catheters remain in the body can help reduce the risk of infection. Condom catheters prevent this problem in men.

If a paralyzed patient lies in any one position for too long, the skin can develop ulcers (also called pressure sores or bedsores), which, though rarely fatal, are extremely painful, costly (bedsores can add an estimated 25 percent to a person's hospital bill because they take a long time to heal), and thoroughly preventable. With the exception of the soles of the feet, human skin cannot tolerate the prolonged pressure of bone against a hard surface. The pressure makes blood platelets stick together, blocking small blood vessels and eventually starving the skin and soft tissues of nutrients. Nurses can and should prevent bedsores by shifting the patient's position every one to two hours and using air mattresses, waterbeds, or foam mattress inserts, which distribute the patient's weight. To stroke patients, even little things make a difference. Be alert for buttons, certain fabrics, and folds in clothing. They irritate the skin. Also, be sure to pad the hard seats of wheelchairs for comfort.

As the medical staff tends to the patient's many needs, they should also explain procedures, solicit and be available to answer questions, and suggest courses of action. The medical staff should explain what caused the stroke and what the potential may be for recovery. And they should explain what the family can do to help.

What should you do if you feel that a loved one isn't getting the care he or she deserves? First of all, don't tolerate second-class treatment. Speak up politely but firmly, and don't take no for an answer.

These are some of the more important criteria that black families can use to ensure that in the early stages of treatment, the patient is receiving an acceptable level of care. Families should keep an eye on these and other points during rehabilitation, which comes after a patient is beyond immediate danger. Chapter 4 discusses this important stage of recovery.

# CHAPTER 4

# Pushing Through Recovery

When Susan Taylor's mother suffered a stroke at the age of eighty, the daughter was privy to two remarkable transformations. The first was shattering. Seeing a formerly independent women confined to a wheelchair, her memory slipping and the right side of her body failing, was nearly too much to bear. "I was devastated," remembers Taylor, editor-in-chief of *Essence* magazine.

But the second change was just as shocking. With considerable willpower and the help of a physical therapist, Taylor's mother progressed from wheelchair to walker to cane, and then her own two feet. Exercising her body and her mind, she recovered bit by bit each day until she had learned to compensate for much of the damage the stroke had wrought. "Now the family can't keep up with her," wrote Taylor.

Her mother's death at the age of eighty-two did little to obscure one central lesson: Black people have always endured. Despite the atrocities of slavery and the continuing legacy of second-class citizenship, African-Americans have ridden the storm with courage and strength.

These qualities can be enormously helpful as black people cope with the aftermath of a stroke. When people suffer a stroke, the world turns inside out. Tasks we take for granted suddenly become formidable; tasks that used to take effort become impossible. Oftentimes, skills we have used every day since childhood—skills like eating, walking, bathing, sitting on a toilet—must be approached differently, and acts that we considered mere afterthoughts the day before a stroke (if we thought about them at all) must be relearned from square one.

Sobering as strokes are, we can all give thanks that patients end up quite differently today than they did a generation or two ago. In the 1950s, stroke survivors typically spent the rest of their lives in wheelchairs. Medical science could do little for them, and therapies for coaxing stroke-damaged nerves and muscles back to life were primitive. Today, if a stroke is nonfatal—and 60 percent of them are—survivors have more of a fighting chance than ever before. From 70 to 90 percent (estimates vary) of people who survive a stroke regain the ability to walk on their own; 50 percent go on to become independent with only minimal assistance; and 30 percent return to normal. In the United States, the average survivor lives for more than seven years after a stroke, and 30 percent survive for eleven years or more.

In some ways, the picture is less bright for the typical African-American patient, for whom stroke presents more medical challenges than for whites. In one study of four hundred mostly black stroke patients at the University Medical Center in Jackson, Mississippi, the average patient survived for five years after the stroke—two fewer years than the national average.

Still, a study at Harlem Hospital Center found that of the nearly 60 percent of stroke patients who were discharged alive, 39 percent were functioning independently with near-normal abilities. Clearly, a stroke is not always hopeless, even in an impoverished black population.

Today's stroke patients gain the benefits of new diagnostic techniques and aggressive rehabilitation therapy. In addition, stroke patients are reaping the fruit of relatively recent discoveries about the recuperative power of the brain. One discovery centers on what doctors call *plasticity*—the ability of the brain to compensate for an injury. Doctors have known for some time that children's brains can adapt to injury, but for years the general wisdom was that adult brains are unforgiving. This theory contributed to the idea that once adults suffered a stroke, there was little hope. But recent evidence suggests that healthy neurons can "sprout" into a stroke-damaged area of the brain and take over some of its former functions. In other cases, the brain figures out ways to circumvent a damaged area. Dr. Paul Bach-y-Rita, chairman of the Department of Rehabilitation Medicine at the University of Wisconsin, Madison, likens the process to what would happen if an earthquake destroyed the phone lines between New York and San Francisco. Initially, it might be impossible to call from one city to the other. After a while, however, someone in California would discover that by calling Denver and asking the operator to connect them with Chicago, and by asking the Chicago operator to connect to New York, a call would get through. The process would be tedious at first, but it would soon speed up as each phone operator along the line became more proficient at transferring calls. This is what Dr. Bachy-Rita and others suspect happens inside the brains of stroke patients. Over time, even in older persons, the brain learns how to adapt.

## WILL THE PATIENT RECOVER?

If the brain's recuperative power were the only consideration, recovery from stroke would be largely an exercise in patience. But there are many other factors at work. We've touched on some of them already. First of all, we know that the likelihood that a stroke will be fatal depends to a great extent on what kind of stroke it is. The probability that the average American will be alive thirty days after the stroke is 80 percent for a cerebral thrombosis, 70 percent for a cerebral embolism, 50 percent for a subarachnoid hemorrhage, and 18 percent for a cerebral hemorrhage (the kind of stroke that's particularly common among African-Americans).

For people who survive the initial incident, the extent of recovery depends on a host of factors. The most important is the degree to which the patient is conscious. Ninety-nine percent of all patients who are comatose when they are admitted to the hospital die within the first five days after the stroke. At the other end of the spectrum, three of every four patients who remain alert after a stroke are still alive three weeks later. Patients who are semiconscious or drowsy have survival rates that fall between these two extremes.

The list below covers other key predictors. For any given item, a good prognosis means a relatively swift or complete recovery. Poor prognosis indicates a negative affect on a patient's rehabilitation, including slower learning and ultimately a less successful recovery. Note that the chances of recovery depend on both the patient's condition and the type of health care he or she receives.

One glance at the table is enough to tell you that the typical black stroke patient has no easy road. Black

### Characteristics of the Patient

| Factor | Good Prognosis | Poor Prognosis |
| --- | --- | --- |
| Ability to balance | No impairment of balance | Persistent difficulty in sitting |
| Ability to follow directions | Ability to follow three-step (though not necessarily verbal) directions | Inability to follow two-step directions |
| Ability to move | Impairment of movement on only one side of the body; normal walking ability | Impaired movement on both sides of the body; inability to walk when discharged from rehabilitation facility |
| Ability to see | No visual problems | Visual problems |
| Ability to speak | No speech problems | Difficulty speaking, especially if patient has difficulty comprehending |
| Age | Younger age | Older age (not a hard-and-fast rule) |
| Behavior | Optimistic attitude; cooperative behavior; acceptance of stroke | Persistent negative attitude and disruptive, uncooperative behavior; denial of stroke |
| Disorientation | Patients who can locate themselves in space or who perveive the world around them | Patients who are disoriented |

## Characteristics of the Patient (*cont.*)

| Factor | Good Prognosis | Poor Prognosis |
|---|---|---|
| Education level | Well educated* | Poorly educated |
| Family | Good support from caring family members; presence of partner | Poor support or absense of family; absense of partner |
| Income | Higher | Lower |
| Incontinence | Regaining bladder | Loss of bladder or and bowel control |
| bowel control for more than four weeks | | within four weeks |
| Intelligence | Normal | Impaired |
| Lifestyle before stroke | Active lifestyle, high degree of motivation | Inactivity, little motivation |
| Mental status | No depression, healthy emotional balance | Depression, inactivity, little motivation, emotional problems |
| Motor activity | Ability to move voluntarily | Inability to move voluntarily |
| Muscle spasms | Moderate or no spasticity | Extremely spastic limbs |
| Muscle tone | Early return of muscle tone after paralysis | Late or no recovery of muscle tone |
| Other diseases | Patients without pre-existing diseases | Patients with hypertension, diabetes, heart disease, arthritis kidney disease, or other illnesses |
| Pain | Little or no pain | Pain in bone or paralyzed muscles |
| Paralysis (duration) | After total paralysis, regaining some movement within three weeks | Total paralysis for longer than three weeks |
| Paralysis (location) | Right side of body | Left side of body |

*Studies also show that highly educated people or those who score high on vocabulary tests often have a poor prognosis, perhaps because the loss of these skills causes depression.

## Characteristics of the Patient (*cont.*)

| Factor | Good Prognosis | Poor Prognosis |
| --- | --- | --- |
| Reflexes | Presence of deep reflexes | Absence of deep reflexes |
| Site of brain damage | Outer tissue | Inner tissue |
| Stroke history | No previous stroke | Previous stroke |
| Unconsciousness | Little or no unconsciousness | Unconsciousness for an extended period of time |

## Characteristics of the Medical Care

| Factor | Good Prognosis | Poor Prognosis |
| --- | --- | --- |
| Eventual residence | A warm, supportive home | Nursing home or other long-term care facility |
| Promptness of initial care | Immediate | Delayed, especially a delay of more than thirty days |
| Quality of care | Continuous nursing care, which minimizes medical complications | Lack of continuous care |
| Rehabilitation site | Comprehensive rehabilitation center | Nursing home |
| Start of rehabilitation after the stroke | Early | Late |

stroke patients are less likely than white patients to be affluent and to have access to expensive comprehensive rehabilitation centers, and they are more likely to have suffered a previous stroke and to have a preexisting disease. In one of the surprisingly few studies of racial differences in stroke recovery, black ischemic patients in Durham, North Carolina, were less alert than white patients upon entering the hospital and recovered more slowly from physical impairment.

Still, the outlook for African-Americans is not completely bleak. As long as preexisting conditions are treated attentively, studies suggest that the mere presence of hypertension, heart disease, or diabetes does not worsen a patient's prognosis. So even though these illnesses increase a person's risk of suffering a stroke, they don't impede recovery from it. That's what doctors found in the Durham study. Black patients had more hypertension and diabetes than did white patients, and they got off to a slower recovery. But three to six months down the road, both black and white patients had regained an average of 90 percent of their physical abilities. In the end, the researchers felt that black patients recovered more slowly because their strokes were more severe.

What's more, one of the traditional strengths of the black community is the way we support each other. Elders look after youngsters; adults care for older relatives; it doesn't take much for close friends to soon become "aunts" and "cousins." This support can be a critical factor in the recovery of a stroke patient, as we will see below. Remember, too, the toughness of spirit that has served African-Americans for generations. This survival skill can help sustain black stroke patients and their families during a long rehabilitation period. The National Institutes of Health is quite clear about the value of courage. When it comes to recuperating from stroke, says NIH, "The most important factor is the will to recover."

The point here is not to alarm but to enlighten. When the odds do not favor us, we must know what we are up against so that we can maximize our chances for full recovery. Knowledge leads to empowerment. Patients and family members who are empowered are less likely to be poorly served by the medical care system and more likely to get the rehabilitation services and care that they want and need.

For example, the medical staff might not give a low-income black patient the same respect that they would a more affluent white patient. When it comes to rehabilitation, family members might receive precious little advice or belated advice; the silence might send the patient and the family the message that rehabilitation would do little good. Yet researchers say that studying the factors that predict the outcome of stroke rehabilitation points to one conclusion. As Dr. Thomas P. Anderson, Clinical Professor of Rehabilitation at Boston University, puts it: "All patients should be given a therapeutic trial of stroke rehabilitation unless they are so ill that they cannot take part in the training program." Studies show that most patients, even those with a poor prognosis, make considerable gains in rehabilitation programs. Knowing this, black stroke patients and their families can push to receive the care that they need.

With this in mind, let's explore in greater detail the mental and physical challenges that stroke patients typically encounter. Then we'll discuss the many ways that these problems can be overcome.

## COMMON MENTAL CHALLENGES

If you were to ask about a person's mental capacity, chances are you would probably mean how smart they are. But mental ability means much more than that. It includes some measure of intelligence, yes, but it also involves a person's ability to pay attention, to remember, to process information, to speak, to read and write, and even to stay awake. All of these functions are controlled by the brain and all can be affected by a stroke.

The location of the stroke determines the mental functions that are disturbed (Figure 12). For example, patients who suffer a stroke in the back of the brain—the so-called *occipital* (ok-sip´-it-al) *lobe*—are frequently forgetful, don't recognize the importance of things they see, and are prone to dementia (mental deterioration). People affected in the lower part of the brain—the *temporal lobe*—are often paranoid and have hallucinations. Patients with strokes in the front of the brain—the *frontal lobe*—can understand and reason just fine. But their personalities change. They can be wildly happy one minute, irritable the next. And they are uninhibited, cracking inappropriate jokes and showing little tact.

A stroke on the right side of the brain affects speech and language, makes it difficult to remember how to do things, and causes the person to be cautious and slow. A stroke on the left side makes it hard to perceive things, causes people to forget language skills, and makes patients impulsive and quick.

To determine the extent of brain damage, doctors use a variety of so-called neuropsychological tests. Asking patients to repeat a sequence of numbers backwards tests memory. Asking the meaning of a proverb (such as "the grass is always greener on the other side") reveals a patient's ability to think abstractly and to solve problems. Showing a patient a design with one section missing and asking him or her to complete the pattern by choosing from among six sections measures nonverbal reasoning skills.

These and many other tests are used for both black and white stroke patients. Yet most of the research

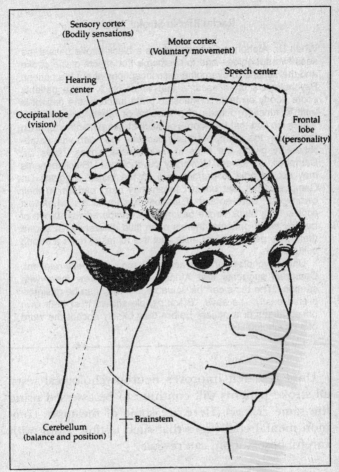

Figure 12. Sections of the brain

that's gone into designing the tests was conducted only with whites. Howard University psychologist Dr. Alphonso Campbell Jr. thinks that was a mistake. (See page 112.)

### Racial Bias in Stroke Tests

When Dr. Alphonso Campbell views a black stroke patient, he sees two struggles—one to overcome the effects of the stroke and the second to overcome misconceptions about the patient. Psychologists often assume that when black stroke patients score poorly on tests to measure brain function, the patient is unfit to function outside of a hospital or rehabilitation facility. "Often we find that the scores of black stroke patients are much lower than the norm, but that's because the norm was established by giving the tests to middle-class whites," says Dr. Campbell, a Howard University psychologist. "Black patients may not be able to perform well on the tests," suggests Dr. Campbell. "But that doesn't mean they can't perform in their own world." Sure enough, Campbell has found that when test scores from black stroke patients are compared with those of healthy black patients, there's often little difference. "It shows that these psychological tests, just like IQ tests, have a strong cultural bias."

Until psychological tests are made more culturally relevant, Campbell suggests that African-Americans view them with caution. "The tests can be valuable, but they can be misinterpreted easily," he says. "Black people should trust their own observations of a patient before they blindly accept the word of a psychologist."

Until research improves neuropsychological tests, all stroke patients will continue to be assessed using the same criteria. Here are some of the more common mental challenges that such testing, along with careful observation, can reveal.

## Impaired Consciousness

Stroke patients vary greatly in level of consciousness. Some are awake and alert, others are comatose, and still others are somewhere in between. Patients may have difficulty paying attention and may be easily distracted. Family members can help by spending time with the patient and being gently supportive. It helps the patient's morale and gives him or her an incentive to get better.

## Memory Problems

Patients may not be able to recall the date or time of day; they may not even remember who they are or where they are. They may be able to remember new information—the name of their doctor or of a medication they are taking—but fail to recall it a few moments later. Long-term memory can be affected as well. Patients may not remember where they went to school or where they were employed before the stroke. Memory problems can be distressing to both patient and family. You can help by trying to take memory lapses in stride and reassuring the patient that healing will come with time.

## Impairment of Higher Mental Function

Ability to solve problems and to use insight and sound judgment may all be impaired. Patients may lose their grasp of common knowledge—the purpose of household appliances, the names of countries, the meaning of traffic signs. They may lose their ability to do arithmetic and to make other calculations. And when presented with two pictures of different objects that have something in common—an overcoat and a pair of socks, for instance—patients may miss the element of similarity. As the brain heals, patients often recover much of this knowledge.

**Loss of Emotional Control**

Some of the more remarkable behavioral changes in stroke patients involve the loss of emotional control. In mild cases, a patient may have a mildly happy or sad thought but end up howling with uncontrollable laughter or sobbing gut-wrenching tears. In more severe cases, the emotion that patients show is the *opposite* of what they feel, so that feeling melancholy triggers peals of laughter. In either case, patients are usually surprised or distressed when observers point out the discrepancy between what they feel inside and what they show others. Some strokes cause severe personality change: without provocation, patients become greatly agitated and confused, and start shouting and swearing. You can help the patient by not being unduly alarmed by the unusual outbursts. The agitation usually passes within a couple of months.

**Fear**

Fear of having a second stroke can make a patient overly cautious or excessively dependent on a caretaker. Many investigations of the aftermath of strokes have studied white patients but not persons of color. One exception is a 1991 survey of 590 ischemic stroke patients hospitalized at New York's Columbia-Presbyterian Medical Center. Researchers there found that about sixteen of every one hundred black patients suffered a second stroke within a year of their first stroke. (This is compared to about eighteen of every one hundred white patients and twelve of every one hundred Hispanic patients.) Another way of looking at these numbers is that for the typical black ischemic stroke patient, the chance of *not* having a second stroke within one year is 84 percent—pretty good odds. After the first year, the risk of stroke generally declines.* Share these statistics with the patient. They may bring a little peace of mind.

## Sexual Problems

Fear of suffering another stroke is one of the many reasons that stroke patients typically curtail their sexual activity. In particular, patients who have endured a hemorrhagic stroke may fear that any activity that raises their blood pressure may cause another. In one survey, men and women of all ages reported less of a sex drive and less frequent intercourse after a stroke. When the researchers asked for specifics, the effects of the stroke were profound. Before their strokes, 43 percent of the women had orgasms and 7 percent reported sexual problems. One year after a stroke, only 11 percent had orgasms, and 48 percent felt they had a sexual problem. As for men, 95 percent had erections, 73 percent ejaculated normally, and none considered themselves to have a sexual problem before their strokes. One year after a stroke, only 38 percent had normal erections, 22 percent ejaculated, and as many as 58 percent thought they had a sexual problem.

---

*The Columbia-Presbyterian researchers discovered that of all of the risk factors they studied, the most accurate predictor of a later stroke was an abnormal initial electrocardiogram (ECG), which increased the risk of later stroke by two to four times. There may be another way to predict a second stroke. Scientists at the Oregon Health Sciences University and the Portland Veterans Administration Center recently announced that a test to measure a certain blood protein called albumin is 75 percent accurate in predicting who will have a second stroke within a year. Low albumin levels are apparently a sign of damage to the blood vessels.

The sexual problems that most stroke patients experience are usually not physical, but psychological. "Patients have a loss of self-esteem, they fear the rejection of their partner, or even abandonment, and are often reluctant to make emotional demands," explains Dr. Murray E. Brandstater, Director of Physical Medicine and Rehabilitation at Loma Linda University Medical Center in California. If you and your stroke-impaired partner have questions about your sexual needs, seek out a caring health professional who can give you supportive counseling. A hospital social worker is a good place to start.

## Denial or Neglect

Strokes hurt the brain's ability to reason, and a stroke patient may deal with the sudden incapacitation by simply denying it exists. Some stroke patients try to resume their normal daily activities, apparently oblivious to their handicaps, and then get frustrated or angry when they cannot. Patients may go so far as to deny that they are blind, even when they plainly cannot see. They may ignore the affected half of their bodies, shaving just half off their beards or dressing on only one side (Figure 13). Patients may go so far as to deny that an affected limb even belongs to them. Dr. Joseph Bleiberg of the Rehabilitation Institute of Chicago remembers one patient who repeatedly refused to acknowledge his paralyzed arm. When the examiner persisted, the patient finally responded, "That's my brother's bad arm. I left my good one home."

Denial is much more common with stroke patients who are affected on the left side of their bodies. It can be overcome, but it takes hard work by the patient, the rehabilitation team, and the family.

## Sensory Impairment

Strokes often have a profound impact on the senses. Our senses take in abundant information about the environment around us. The nerves relay the information to the brain, which processes it. In stroke patients, a link along this well-rehearsed sensory chain is broken. The senses may be delivering messages to a brain that cannot process them. Patients may be able to see objects only within a certain area in their normal field of vision. Experienced cooks may repeatedly ruin meals because their minds cannot process the aromatic cues that food is burning. Patients may not recognize a familiar object like a bell or an apple placed before their eyes or into their hand, even though their senses (vision, hearing, smell, taste, touch) work perfectly fine. Or they may not recognize a familiar face, even the face of their spouse or child. This condition, known as *agnosia* (ag-no´-see-ah), is similar to *anomia* (eh-no´-me-ah)—the inability to name things. Sensory impairment can be alarming; not recognizing the face of a family member whom the patient has known for a lifetime is disturbing to both parties. Without the spark of recognition, a hospitalized patient feels surrounded in a strange place by strangers. And the family can feel detached from their loved one at a vulnerable, anxious time.

## Impairment of Learned Movements

Some stroke patients have fully functional senses and normal muscles. But when handed a toothbrush,

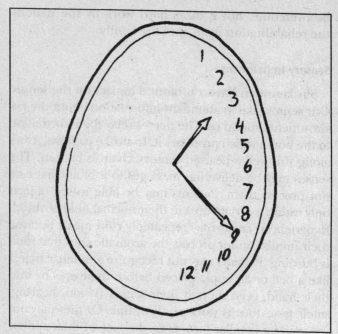

Figure 13. A clock drawn by a stroke patient

they don't know what to do with it. Or when presented with a musical instrument, an accomplished musician won't be able to pick out the simplest tune. These patients suffer from *apraxia*—the inability to perform learned movements. Patients with *ideomotor apraxia* might perform an action spontaneously but be unable to do so on demand. Those with *ideational apraxia* cannot perform tasks that involve a sequence of steps, such as answering a doorbell, looking through a peephole, and opening a door. With *dressing apraxia*, a patient who is handed a folded scarf or shirt will not know how to put it on. Dressing apraxia is often persistent, but apraxia in general can improve as a patient repeatedly learns and practices various movements—an exercise families can help with.

## Speech Disorders

Speech disorders are common. Some stroke patients speak quite freely but distort their words into a stream of meaningless syllables. Others slur their speech or speak with great hesitation, choosing each word painstakingly. Some patients have *speech apraxia,* an inability to program otherwise functional muscles to speak.

Many patients with stroke-induced speech disorders have difficulty understanding spoken and written words, and whether orally or in writing, can't seem to find the words to express themselves. This condition, known as *aphasia* (ah-fa´-zha), is a widespread problem; more severe forms of the disorder affect upwards of twenty thousand stroke patients each year. Many who have experienced it say it is the most psychologically devastating of all of the effects of stroke.

Patients with aphasia typically substitute one word for another. Friends and family of Lillian Washington,* a black grandmother who suffered a stroke, recall that she would often say the word "chicken" when asked to identify a picture of any familiar object (a hat, for example) that her mind could not readily name. Immediately she would realize her mistake, telling them with mild annoyance, *"That's* not a chicken." But her brain had beaten her to the answer.

Aphasia comes in many forms. Mrs. Washington had *semantic aphasia,* in which the substituted word belongs in the same family as the intended word. In

---

*Not her real name.

*acoustic aphasia,* the patient substitutes a word that sounds like the intended word (for example, "mat" for "hat"). With *global aphasia,* a person can manage only a single utterance over and over ("youyou-youyou").

Speech therapy is a standard practice for patients with aphasia. Admittedly, aphasia is such a complex disorder that researchers disagree over whether speech therapy does any good. As one prominent neurologist commented twenty years ago, "The classic aphasic patient comes in on a stretcher and isn't talking. When he leaves, he is walking but not talking." But in one of the few investigations of the effectiveness of speech therapy, a 1986 study of ischemic stroke patients who scored poorly on a standardized speech test called PICA (the Porch Index of Communicative Ability) improved significantly after receiving eight to ten hours of treatment each week by a speech pathologist for twelve weeks during the first six months following the stroke. Another study of aphasic patients found that those who received treatment performed much better than untreated patients when it came to speaking, reading comprehension, spelling, and other skills. Both individual and group therapy helps. Patients have been known to improve in speech and language as many as six to seven years after a stroke, so the watchwords are patience, persistence, and hope.

In general, one of the key factors in relearning to speak seems to be timing: the earlier therapy starts, the more the patient recovers. The brain seems to regain its speech skills spontaneously for about the first six months after a stroke. One of the reasons that researchers endorse therapy is the finding that, with therapy, many improvements can occur for as long as

## Aphasic Patients Talk Back

For family and friends, helping a loved one who has aphasia can be a confusing, frustrating ordeal. But what is it like for the stroke patient? Dr. Madge Skelly, professor of communication disorders at St. Louis University Graduate School, posed that question to fifty recovered aphasic patients. The responses reveal much about how medical staff and family members alike can treat aphasic patients more humanely and hasten their recovery.

- Assume that the patient can understand you even if they're unresponsive. In the survey, every patient stressed that they comprehended much more than they were given credit for. It was just hard to get the words out.
- Speak slowly, but avoid talking down to the patient. Aphasics said that nearly everyone talked too fast. One patient said normal speech sounded like an audio tape played at high speed.
- Don't ask too many questions at once. With aphasia, even repeating a question can interrupt a patient's processing a response. "My wheels go round a great deal slower now," remarked one patient. "But nobody seems to know this but me."
- Be patient. Patients were quick to note sighs of frustration, drumming of fingers, and other signs of impatience, which hurt their morale and progress.
- Be quiet. Noise is destructive to aphasic patients. One commented that the steady drone of televisions, loudspeaker announcements, and other routine hospital noise was "worse than the airport." Aphasics need peace to help sort the confusion in their minds.
- Respect the patient's intelligence. Being asked to recite the alphabet or being shown pictures or storybooks obviously meant for children was degrading, and the authoritarian attitudes of some psychological testers was off-putting to patients. Family members can help, too: just treat the patient the way you would like to be treated if the tables were turned.

a year—far past the six-month point. The therapist may use several different techniques to help a patient, including oral drills, sung sentences, the use of gestures to augment the spoken word, practice in constructing sentences, exercises in matching objects with pictures—and lots of encouragement. With the support of her family and friends, who tutored her with flashcards of objects and encouraged her return to health, Mrs. Washington eventually regained her language skills.

One of the newer therapeutic developments for aphasics is a computer program that helps patients learn to communicate. The program, called Computerized Visual Communication (C-VIC), displays on a Macintosh computer screen any of three hundred flash-card images, including household goods, food, body parts, clothes, and photographs of people the patient knows. The images also include symbols for prepositions and verbs, such as outstretched hands for "want." By using the computer's "mouse" to select images in a certain sequence, a patient can string together a simple sentence, such as "I want hat." Dr. Michael Weinrich, a neurologist at Baltimore's Kernan Hospital and the inventor of C-VIC, says the device seems to stimulate even severely aphasic patients to begin to vocalize sentences of their own. "We found an impressive improvement in the performance of patients," Dr. Weinrich told the *Washington Post*.

## Depression

Depression affects as many as 30 to 60 percent of stroke patients, by one estimate, and some researchers believe treatment of depression is stroke patients' single most unmet need. Depressed patients may be withdrawn, irritable, or anxious, and may devote unusual attention to their sleep habits and other mundane matters. With their bodies, lives, emotions, and very thoughts suddenly thrown into a spiraling chaos, patients may even suspect they are going mad.

The reasons for depression are not difficult to understand. Frequently the loss of physical and mental ability is catastrophic and overwhelming. Formerly self-sufficient patients can find themselves completely dependent on others. Blacks and other people of color may not have access to the best medical and rehabilitation facilities. Young patients may not have set aside enough money to afford ideal care. Elderly patients whose spouses have died and whose children have moved away may find themselves with little family support.

Depression can do more than affect a patient's mental outlook. It can also affect their recovery. Dr. Thomas R. Price and his colleagues at the University of Maryland School of Medicine say that while stroke patients generally get better over time, whether or not they are depressed, patients who are depressed do not improve as quickly. When Price surveyed sixty-three mostly low-income stroke patients—about half of them black—released from the university's hospital, he found that depressed patients had significantly more trouble managing routine daily activities (walking, dressing, eating, speaking, etc.) even two years after the stroke. Lack of awareness by health professionals hurts, too. "[Doctors] don't diagnose it, and don't really expect it," says Dr. Price. Instead, doctors and families often wait in vain for the patient to improve, eventually giving up hope.

Depression is a normal part of the aftermath of any disability. Immediately after a stroke hits, patients experience shock, which they typically show as anxiety and feelings of hopelessness. Then they go through a stage of denial, when their anxiety diminishes but the hopelessness remains. Depression sets in during the early stages of recovery, and is typically most severe between six months and two years following the stroke. The extent of the depression also depends on the type of stroke. One study of low-income black patients found that the more toward the front of the brain stroke damage is located, the more depressed a patient is prone to be. Families may notice bitterness, withdrawal, or any number of changes that may be uncharacteristic of the patient. As the patient adjusts to the disability and gradually gains mastery over it, depression recedes.

Depression can last for months, but it can be eased with the reassurance, support, and encouragement of the medical team and family members. Psychotherapy from a supportive counselor can help. Stroke clubs (support groups of stroke patients) can help, too. (See Appendix B for information on stroke clubs.) Severe cases can be successfully treated with antidepressant medication. One such drug, nortriptyline, has been shown helpful in preliminary tests with stroke patients at Johns Hopkins University. Psychiatrist Dr. John R. Lipsey, who headed the study, told *Science News* that while some depressions in stroke patients benefit from psychotherapy, "we think the majority are due to chemical imbalances in the brain." Medication can correct these imbalances.*

---

*Ironically, certain medicines for depression can cause behavioral changes themselves. Tricyclic medications, a large class of antidepres-

## COMMON PHYSICAL CHALLENGES

Some of the most obvious and dramatic effects of a stroke are physical—a leg that abruptly collapses, a hand or arm that suddenly turns numb. Stroke patients can lose their reflexes, so that the classic tap below the kneecap that usually triggers an automatic leg-kick brings no reaction at all. Even touching a patient's eye may not make them blink. Often the face alone reveals the telltale signs of a stroke; one side loses muscle control, and so half of a normally symmetrical face—one eyelid, one cheek, one corner of the mouth—droops. Without control of the tongue, patients may not be able to swallow, and eating becomes a formidable challenge. Without sure control of the lips or the sphincter muscles of the bladder, patients face the indignity of drooling mouths and soiled underclothing.

A stroke can cause any bodily function that's controlled by nerves and muscles—and there are many—to fail. To understand why, consider what normally happens when a person moves a muscle. When an ice cream vendor hands you a cone, you reach out to accept it without thinking. Reaching for an item that we want is a skill that we master in early childhood. But behind this seemingly simple task is a symphony of messages and movement. Muscles need orders to

---

sants, can make a patient confused. Treatment of other emotional and physical disorders can trigger certain behavioral changes as well. Anticholinergic drugs, which are given for anxiety, nausea, heart disorders, ulcers, and other conditions, can cause confusion and agitation. Sleeping pills, diuretics, antihistamines, and other medicines may cause unwanted behavioral effects. Doctors should be alert for these changes, but patients and their families should be, too. The side effects can be minimized by reducing dosages or switching to other medications.

move, and the directions come from the brain (and sometimes the spinal cord). When our eyes spot the ice cream cone, our brain sends a stream of instructions through our spinal cord to the muscles of the shoulder, arm, and hand. The messages travel through *motor nerves* that are strung end to end like telephone wires. In fact, the messages themselves are tiny electrical impulses that the muscles translate into specific commands, like "bend your elbow" or "open your hand." As the muscles that control the elbow dutifully push or pull the arm bones, other nerves—*sensory nerves*—measure the position of the elbow and relay the information back to the brain. That's why you can close your eyes and still know whether or not your elbow is bent or your hand is open.

So the nerves function as a communications link, relaying commands from the brain to hundreds of muscles and simultaneously sending back a steady flow of information that lets the brain monitor how well its instructions are being carried out. If something happens to the brain, the nervous system loses its command post. Like a telephone network with no operator to place or receive calls, incoming and outgoing messages never reach their destination. The body's control over one of the most basic aspects of life—motion—has shut down. This explains why stroke patients can lose control of their muscles and can even lose the sensations of pain, pressure, and cold.

Most of us scarcely give our nerves much thought, even though they are critical to our day-to-day functioning. *Cranial nerves* are a case in point. We take for granted these nerves that serve the facial muscles, the eyes, the ears, and the mouth. But these important nerves control the muscles that enable us to look in a certain direction, open and close our eyes, and focus our vision; smile and purse our lips; and chew and swallow. A stroke can make these tasks difficult or impossible.

A stroke's effect on the rest of the muscles of the body can vary. Our brains are divided into hemispheres, with the left half of the brain controlling the right half of the body, and vice versa. A stroke in the left hemisphere can leave the entire right side of the body numb and paralyzed. (Oddly, strokes most often affect the right side of the brain, which controls the left half of the body.) One patient recalled that after his stroke, his left arm and hand were a "baffling puzzle. They were there, but they also weren't. When I grasped my left hand with my right, it felt like a piece of soft, warm lead."

Sometimes strokes cause a patient's arm or leg to tense in a rigid spasm as nerve messages that normally signal the muscles to relax become confused. Doctors call these spasms *contractures*. A patient may not be able to easily move the affected limb, which can become seized by the muscles to the point of distortion. When this happens, muscle coordination is severely compromised. About 80 percent of patients find that certain actions trigger involuntary movements in a stroke-affected area. For example, yawning or stretching a normal arm may inadvertently raise the paralyzed arm. The first time they occur, patient and family often take these involuntary movements to mean a sudden sign of progress. But they are simply an unusual effect of the brain disturbance caused by the stroke.

A stroke can cause the muscles of an affected limb to deteriorate from disuse. After as little as a week in bed, the lack of constant movement that keeps normal muscles in tone causes tissue to begin to waste away, and once-firm muscles become flabby. Muscle tone improves as a stroke-damaged limb begins to heal and as physical therapy starts to put dormant muscles through their paces.

Stroke patients are often paralyzed in their upper extremities—more frequently, in fact, than in their legs. But flaccid shoulder muscles may be too weak to support a patient's weight when sitting up in bed or even to support the arm when a patient is standing. As a result, the shoulder can become dislocated. To avoid this, make sure the patient wears an arm sling when walking about. Also, use pillows in the patient's bed to prop up the paralyzed arm. These give the shoulder adequate support until muscle tone returns.

## THE ROAD TO REHABILITATION

The goal in recovering from stroke is to try to regain the level of health and ability to function that the patient had before the stroke and to prevent more strokes from occurring, all while helping the patient cope with a new and unfamiliar body in a new and sometimes frightening world. That can be a tall order, considering the many impairments that a patient is up against. But just as strokes show the frightening devastation of sudden brain impairment, they also demonstrate the remarkable capacity of the human body and mind to bounce back.

As a rule, the mental and behavioral changes brought by a stroke begin to fade in the first few months following a stroke, as the brain slowly recovers its bearings. It is here that the brain shows its plastic-

---

**Quiet Misery for Stroke Patients**

It may not be one of the more talked about complications of stroke, but it can make life miserable. Constipation is a quiet frustration in many stroke patients. A stroke doesn't usually impair the bowel, but prolonged inactivity does. It slows the movement of food through the intestines. Standard hospital food, which is typically low in fiber, doesn't help. Certain medicines can also cause constipation, among them diuretics (which are frequently given for hypertension). Constipation is also one of the many signs of depression. Constipation can be prevented or overcome by eating plenty of fiber-rich fruits, vegetables, and bran; giving a patient plenty to drink (six to eight glasses of liquids daily); and encouraging him to be as mobile as possible, doctor's orders permitting.

---

ity. Some researchers believe that the brain continues to heal even after a year, so it's important for stroke patients and their families not to give up hope if change seems slow in coming. In the meantime, stroke researchers advise stimulating patients to encourage the return of mental health and to help ward off the sense of isolation. Once neuropsychological tests identify how a stroke has affected a patient, therapists can work with patients first to help them become aware of the problem and then to figure out how to compensate for it.

There are many ways to encourage a sluggish, stroke-damaged brain to heal. The traditional approach is to use occupational therapy—teaching a patient to perform menial and then progressively more complex tasks. The idea is that by learning to tie a shoe or unlock a door, patients simultaneously learn to reason, solve problems, remember information, and master more sophisticated challenges. More recent strategies of stroke rehabilitation focus on teach-

ing these skills directly. Some therapists use psychoneurological tests themselves as training tools to help
patients regain lost skills. Some, like aphasia expert Dr.
Michael Weinrich, use computers, which can give a patient instant feedback and colorful, positive reinforce-
ment—and an automatic record of the patient's
progress.

The recovery of lost motor skills starts to take place
within a matter of days or even hours. Reflexes start to
reappear. Mobility begins to return. Muscle tone improves. In anywhere from the first week to the first
month, the first voluntary movement appears. Patients
learn how to move the muscles first in a group, then
more selectively. The large muscles of the leg recover
first, then the arm, then the fine muscles of the hands
and fingers. Eventually many patients who could initially do little more than lie motionless in bed learn to
roll over, then maneuver into a sitting position, then
hoist themselves into a wheelchair. Clumsiness gives
way to finesse. Range of motion returns to the joints.
Over the course of six months to a year, patients slowly
regain their lost skills.

Family members can play a valuable role in this
process from the very beginning, and should volunteer their services as soon as they can summon the
strength to do so. For example, massaging the muscles
and starting range-of-motion exercises from day one
can help minimize the effects of contractures even before formal physical therapy begins.

One important role for the family is helping a patient eat comfortably. Eating is often challenging for
stroke patients. Strokes can damage nerves of the
tongue and jaw, causing lack of coordination and an
inability to feel food in the mouth. The muscles of the

tongue and lips may be weak. Thus chewing and swallowing can be difficult.

To help patients who have trouble chewing, be sure to offer very tender (not stringy) meats, fish with the bones removed, and vegetables that have been thoroughly cooked (no longer crisp) but not mushy. Stroke patients who have difficulty swallowing are at risk of choking. You can help by avoiding certain foods that are difficult to move around the mouth and swallow: dry or crisp foods, peanut butter, finely pureed or mashed foods, bananas. Avoid tart or excessively sweet juices, which aggravate drooling. If a patient's mouth is dry from reduced salivation, try to moisten foods to make it easier to move food in the mouth. And make sure the patient drinks plenty of liquids daily.

Often one of the more unexpected mealtime challenges is helping a patient maintain interest in a meal. Poor short-term memory and poor vision may make a patient depressed or disinterested in eating. Cheerfulness and patience go a long way in helping a patient recover. Finally, when planning a diet for a stroke patient, be sure to ask a doctor about the interaction between food and the patient's medication. Some dietary choices improve the effectiveness of certain medicines, and you may want to incorporate these foods into the patient's diet.

Patients whose improvement begins within four weeks after the stroke recover more fully than do those whose recovery takes longer to begin. Some patients reach a plateau where further improvement slows to a stop. This is particularly true when strokes involve the hand, which often recovers only 20 to 30 percent or so of its former function. In other patients, recovery approaches 100 percent.

How fast and how completely a given patient recovers depends on a number of factors. One is the body's inherent ability to heal, an ability that changes over time. Again, improvements occur rapidly at first and slow in subsequent months. Patients can continue to make significant gains six months to a year or longer after a stroke, but the rate of recovery is more gradual.

The second factor is the severity of the problem. Slight injuries heal much faster with fewer lingering effects than do more severe ones.

Third, recovery depends on the emotional and psychological makeup of the patient. "Two individuals with very similar deficits may differ greatly in their degree of disability," advises Dr. Murray E. Brandstater of Loma Linda University. "A patient with minimal left hemiparesis [slight paralysis] may function very poorly and require considerable assistance, while another patient with left hemiplegia [full paralysis] may learn to compensate well and become independent."

This is where a patient's emotional toughness and will to recover play an enormous role. Recovering lost mental and motor skills is hard work. It takes regular practice day in and day out, over a period of many months, and progress can be agonizingly slow. The patient's confidence and sense of self must be gently nurtured despite frequent self-doubt and despair. In the earliest stages of rehabilitation, a patient's most diligent efforts to talk or walk or even move a paralyzed limb may be fruitless, causing frustration, anxiety—and the doubly distressing realization that the patient can do little to relieve the anxiety. In the face of mountainous obstacles, it takes a great deal not to give up. For black patients, the ability to summon an inner strength—the same source of fortitude and

pride that has sustained the race to the present day—
is key.

Fourth, recovery depends on the timing of rehabilitation. The sooner rehabilitation begins, the greater
the recovery will eventually be.

Fifth, recovery depends on the type of rehabilitation
program that the patient enters. Some patients receive
rehabilitation on the medical ward to which they are
admitted in the hospital, but this is an unlikely setting
for receiving the sustained attention that stroke patients need because the medical staff is often busy tending to the needs of more critically ill patients. Nursing
homes provide some rehabilitation services, but their
expertise and commitment to stroke patients is often
limited. One of the best settings is a special stroke rehabilitation unit that provides comprehensive care from
the early stages of stroke to discharge, including follow-
up. Studies show that patients who receive such contin-
uous care enjoy much fuller recovery than do others;
from 60 to 90 percent of patients at comprehensive rehabilitation programs are well enough to be sent home
(as opposed to being sent to a long-term care facility
such as a nursing home) once they are discharged.

Finally, the speed and extent of recovery also depend
on how aggressive the therapy is. In years past, doctors
didn't understand that the human body could recover
from a stroke. As a result, rehabilitation programs were
never a routine part of care of these patients, and recovery was sharply limited. For example, if stroke-impaired
patients had difficulty walking, they often showed the
classic signs of a twisted, deformed leg and brief, awk-
ward steps—without much prospect for improvement.
Modern rehabilitation techniques have changed all of
that. Today, a stroke patient who gets aggressive therapy

## The Team Approach to Rehabilitation

Stroke patients are typically aided by a team of health professionals, each with a different role. This team approach is so beneficial for patients that American hospitals and rehabilitation centers must employ it in order to be accredited. Each team need not employ every health professional listed here, and any given stroke patient does not necessarily need the help of each person. To an extent, some team members can help assume the responsibilities of others; in the absence of a speech therapist, for example, nurses can help an aphasic patient by speaking simply, speaking to the patient as an adult rather than talking down, and accepting the patient's best efforts rather than correcting errors. Here is a breakdown of a typical team along with a brief explanation of each person's role.

A *physician* orders and interprets diagnostic tests, prescribes medication and feeding, arranges for surgery if needed, and generally oversees the patient's recovery.

*Nurses* provide twenty-four-hour bedside care, taking vital signs (blood pressure, pulse, etc.), turning the patient in bed, and helping the patients control and regulate their bladder and bowels. Nurses help a patient perform range-of-motion exercises and help patients begin to regain their mobility.

A *physical therapist's* job is to help patients regain the ability to move and function. Physical therapists help patients recover the balance and muscle control needed to walk. They also help stroke-impaired parts of the body recover strength, flexibility, and range of motion, while they help the patient compensate by using parts of the body that are unaffected by the stroke.

An *occupational therapist* helps patients with many of the same skills covered by a physical therapist. The focus here, though, is relearning the skills that patients need to dress, eat, wash, comb their hair, brush their teeth, use the toilet, and other activities of daily living (often referred to as "ADL"). The goal is to achieve a comfortable daily mix of work, rest, play, and sleep.

*Speech therapists* evaluate speech disorders and help patients express themselves orally. They also help patients improve their reading and writing skills as well as their ability to comprehend what they hear. Speech therapists help other members of the medical team and family members understand how to best communicate with a stroke patient and teach ways to stimulate the recovery of speaking skills.

*Vocational counselors* can evaluate a patient with an eye toward returning to work and can suggest rehabilitation tools to best prepare a patient for the workplace. Vocational counselors can also help with job placement.

Other counselors, including *psychotherapists,* help patients and family members adjust to the emotional and psychological burden of stroke. *Social service workers* assess the needs and resources of the family and patient and find resources within the community to help satisfy those needs.

The *family* and *patient* are part of the rehabilitation team, too. Together, they can help set realistic goals and work diligently together to meet them.

## What to Look for in a Rehabilitation Facility

Once a stroke patient is past the point of immediate danger and can be released from the hospital, a discharge planner, working closely with the patient's physician, should visit with family and patient and discuss options for rehabilitation. "If no one comes to you to explain what lies ahead, speak up," advises Thelma Edwards, director of program development at the National Stroke Association. Rehabilitation can occur in a number of settings, including nursing homes, skilled-nursing facilities, outpatient clinics, free-standing rehabilitation units, and even in the patient's home. Ask the discharge planner to recommend the best way to give the patient optimal care. If she or he mentions several rehabilitation options, remember that the quality of care in these settings has a great deal to do with how quickly and completely the patient recovers. Here are some questions that can help you evaluate any given rehabilitation facility:

1. Does the program include psychoneurological tests as well as physical therapy? The testing reveals the precise functional and cognitive abilities and skills that the patient lacks. Once these deficits are known, therapists can work on helping the patient remedy them. But leaping into therapy without understanding what is wrong with the patient risks overlooking some of the patient's less obvious needs.

2. Is the program affiliated with a university? Rehabilitation centers that operate under the auspices of a university medical center often use the most modern techniques and have access

to up-to-date information. Sometimes these centers even develop treatments for stroke patients.

3.    Are the health care providers licensed? Most families prefer
to have a stroke victim cared for by the nearest health professionals. For African-Americans, this may mean choosing from
among therapists who may operate unconventional practices, including some from within their homes. You can check on the cre-
dentials of any provider by asking if they are licensed to operate.
Most states use licensing boards to try to achieve a uniform
standard of therapy. There are plenty of excellent health care
professionals—African-Americans and whites alike—who aren't
affiliated with universities, but every good health care provider
should be operating under a state license, and should be able to
produce the license if you ask to see it.

4.    Are the providers members of national professional organizations? A number of national groups strive to maintain profes-
sionalism and continuing education for their members. For
example, physical therapists have the American Physical Therapy Association; speech therapists have the American Speech,
Language, and Hearing Association; and occupational therapists have the American Occupational Therapy Association. Ask
your health providers if they belong to any national professional
organizations. If they're good at their jobs and they take rehabilitation seriously, chances are they do.

can stretch the body's recuperative powers to the ut-
most. With mechanical aids (ankle braces, special
shoes) and corrective surgery when appropriate, stroke
patients often learn to walk again. In fact, various experts estimate that today's stroke patients face a 70 to
95 percent likelihood of learning to walk independently, providing they receive proper rehabilitation.

## FAMILY INVOLVEMENT

One of the most crucial ingredients in recovery
from stroke is the role of the family. In fact, Dr. Paul

Bach-y-Rita goes so far as suggesting that having a supportive family is the single most important factor in recovery. "The sensitive, persistent input of family members can be of the highest importance in the rehabilitation of the stroke patient, and can even lead to a high degree of recovery without professional rehabilitation." These are important words for black patients who may not live near a good rehabilitation facility or may lack the money to pay for expert care.

Family members understand how a patient managed to overcome previous obstacles and know what sorts of motivation and support are most effective. Visits from family members can help minimize a patient's sense of isolation and fear, and family members can take an active role in physical rehabilitation, which must be pursued daily for best results. Family members can be indispensable providers of emotional support, giving warmth and comfort in times of distress. One study shows that stroke patients who have partners recover much more quickly and completely from a stroke than do patients without partners, perhaps because these (and other) family members can help discourage negative habits and motivate patients to increase their activity. For patients with neither partners nor other family members, friends and to some extent even pets can be enormously helpful in providing support, encouragement, and companionship.

Family members have needs, too. Figuring out ways to provide for the many needs of a suddenly handicapped family member can be formidable, and the challenge can be even greater if the family does not function well to begin with or if the stricken member is the family's traditional decision-maker. Families may have to adjust to very different routines, a sense of social isolation, and lack of sleep. Depending on the health of the patient, they may have to get used to anything from occasional errands to twenty-four-hour bedside care. Their own health may suffer as they devote more and more time to helping the patient recover. In families unable to afford to pay a caretaker for the patient—and that includes many black families—the family member who becomes the primary caretaker may have to give up his or her job. This can have important financial implications for the family. There's no doubt that, as one rehabilitation specialist—himself a former stroke patient—put it, "A stroke is actually a family illness."

Families of severely disabled patients typically undergo three stages of adjustment, according to Grady Bray, a psychologist who studied sixty families of severely disabled patients at the Georgia Warm Springs Hospital and Georgia Rehabilitation Center. In the *anxiety stage,* families move from fearing a loved one's death to confronting the painful reality of the new handicap. During this stage, families often show their anxiety by being obsessed with and being critical of the competence of the medical staff, even as they fear that criticism may mean that the patient receives worse care. Denial of the patient's illness is common at this stage. During the *acceptance stage,* families take an active role in helping the patient recover. They are now receptive to medical advice and may criticize the team for not offering it earlier—not realizing that their own denial prevented them from hearing the same advice when the medical team tried to talk with the family earlier. In the *assimilation stage,* families make more lasting adjustments to accommodate the patient's disabilities.

Family members need to be educated about stroke and what the patient is going through. They need to know how to adjust to the patient's condition and what to expect in the days and months ahead. They need to understand the danger of becoming over-protective to the point that the patient becomes overly dependent on them and fails to make progress. Counseling can be helpful, especially with support groups of other families of stroke patients.

## NURTURING THE SPIRIT

A strong spiritual base helps family and patient cope with the aching questions and uncertainties that strokes inevitably bring. (Will he die? Does she know what is happening to her? He can't talk; can he understand me? And even: how could God do this to us?) Whether it adheres to the tenets of organized religion or follows a more individual course of meditation and reflection, being grounded in a form of spirituality can help people place a stroke in a larger context and help them find answers.

Here again, the African-American community benefits from its historical reliance on religion. For generations, the church has been central in the lives of black Americans. Even before white missionaries and the slave trade introduced Africans to Christianity, African religions provided direction in times of confusion and comfort in times of distress. Today, this same sense of spiritual connection helps African-Americans find support and reassurance in the difficult aftermath of a stroke.

In darker moments, it helps to remember that a stroke is different from many other serious illnesses.

Unlike Alzheimer's disease, advanced cancer, and other chronic conditions that cause patients to slowly deteriorate, a stroke that is not immediately fatal offers the promise of at least limited recovery. The onset of stroke is sudden, but patients generally do not worsen. Most of those who survive the initial event get better, to one extent or another, and some recover virtually all of their lost abilities.

## WORDS TO HEAL BY

On the whole, although the physical and emotional impact of stroke can be long-lasting, the prospects for a typical patient are nowhere near as dim as they were a generation ago. Up to 50 percent of the patients who survive a stroke are eventually able to lead fully independent lives, and up to 80 percent gain a degree of self-sufficiency that allows them to function capably with only minor assistance at home. Thirty percent of surviving patients even return to work. Only two of every ten stroke patients are so gravely impaired by the end of a rehabilitation program that they must be institutionalized.

Recovery takes persistence. It also demands flexibility to adapt to new circumstances. Patients may have to get used to a vastly different life—dressing and bathing with one hand, wearing a strange leg brace, handling curious looks from strangers. Those who can summon the courage to continue on, despite disappointment, depression, and pain, recover the fullest.

# CHAPTER 5

# Prevention Is
# the Best Medicine

In the red-clay hills of Georgia, a mother and her child walk hand in hand to a clinic that might save his young life. The boy has sickle cell anemia, and doctors are anxious to measure the blood flow to his brain. Holding a small probe to his temple, the examiners send ultrasound waves painlessly through the boy's head. They look for telltale changes in the sound waves that warn that the boy's abnormally shaped red blood cells have partially blocked an artery—a sign of a future stroke. If they know their young patient is at risk, the doctors can act today to help prevent the stroke from happening tomorrow. And that will give the youngster a better chance of having a normal, happy life.

Twenty years ago, the average sickle cell patient died in adolescence. Today, many patients live into their forties. In the not-too-distant future, sickle cell patients may have an even shot at a normal lifespan. If so, prevention will be a key element.

None of us ever wants to be sick. But on the other hand, let's face it: when black Americans set personal priorities, disease prevention doesn't rank very high on the list. How can we afford to see a doctor when it's hard enough to make the rent every month? Who has time to exercise when we're scrambling to keep a job? Who can be concerned about problems that might happen down the road when our children need food and clothing and good schools *now*?

We give lots of reasons for letting our health slip by the wayside. What we often don't realize is that there are even better reasons to take care of ourselves.

First of all, staying healthy can help us meet the challenges that face us every day. Eating sensibly helps us control the things we can see (like our waistline) as well as things we can't (like blood pressure and cholesterol). And that can help us be more comfortable in the world. Taking time to get centered by meditating, reading, or taking a leisurely stroll can lend us the peace of mind it takes to handle the more stressful demands that are placed on our shoulders. Making a habit of exercising regularly, whether by walking, jogging, swimming, aerobics, basketball, or any number of other activities, helps relax us as it increases our stamina and gives us energy to make it through the day.

Our health is also one part of our lives that we can control. That's important, because many of the stresses that African-Americans face are beyond our ability to change. We can't change racist attitudes. We can't change the way that white men split apart generations of black families on the auction block and then accused black parents of not being able to keep their families together. We can't stop folks from claiming we are incapable of learning, despite the fact that many of our children attend marginal schools, and for many years laws forbade teaching blacks to read. We can't prevent people from accusing us of laziness at a time when corporations are taking precious jobs from low-income communities and replacing them with toxic waste dumps.

But we *can* take charge of our health. When we stay on our medication, and watch what we eat, and exercise regularly, and have regular checkups, we give ourselves a gift that no one can take away. And we share that gift with our loved ones, too. Our children, who rely on us for guidance and support and love, need parents with sound minds and bodies. Our friends and families all benefit when we take good care of ourselves.

One of the smartest reasons for staying healthy is that a little effort now pays off tremendously down the road. Thanks in part to better prevention, millions of people who would have died from strokes during the next twenty-five years *won't* die at all. That's according to a 1991 study by the nonprofit Batelle Medical Technology Assessment and Policy Research Center in Columbus, Ohio. Batelle analysts wondered about the future of stroke, so they asked physicians, scholars, and government scientists to estimate how many stroke patients would die if the current death rate continues for the next twenty-five years. The answer: 5.1 million people. Then they asked how many patients would die if people live more healthful lifestyles and medical researchers come up with better medicines and medical procedures. This time, the answer was only 2.9 million—nearly half of the former number. Of the 2.1 million people who will be spared fatal strokes, an estimated 10 percent will be helped by new medical procedures. Another 40 percent will benefit from advancements in drug therapy. But the largest number of lives—50 percent of the total—will be saved because people take better care of themselves.

So it pays to take preventive measures. That may sound like money. Admittedly, at a time when an estimated thirty-seven million Americans have no health insurance, gaining access to affordable health care is becoming more and more difficult, especially for African-Americans, who are disproportionately poor. But it's far less costly to prevent an illness than to treat it once it develops. Besides, much of what we can do to prevent strokes is free. Eating less salt and jogging around the neighborhood don't cost a cent, but they can lower our blood pressure and reduce our risk of stroke. Seeing a doctor regularly and taking medication to reduce hypertension can cost money, but having a stroke costs much more. "It costs an estimated $300 to $2,000 a year for the medications needed to keep high blood pressure under control, depending on the number of drugs the doctor prescribes and the cost of those medications," explains hypertension expert Dr. Neil Shulman of Emory University. On the other hand, "Nursing home care for victims of stroke costs in the range of $25,000 to $30,000 a year." Even for people who don't need a nursing home, the cost of hospitalization after a stroke can be devastating. In 1996, the average cost of a hospital stay after a stroke stood at $18,244.

Finally, there are good medical reasons to prevent a stroke. Despite the many advances of modern medicine, strokes still claim thousands of lives and thousands of additional cases of disability each year. Despite its marvelous plasticity, our brains are still vulnerable organs that are clearly susceptible to long-term injury. "The central nervous system is unique in its complexities but unforgiving when damaged," suggests Dr. W. Neath Folger, a neurologist with the Mayo

## Where Does God's Will Enter the Picture?

It's natural to be troubled about aspects of illness that we don't understand. Why do strokes strike some young people in their prime, while leaving many elders untouched? Why do some patients recover while leaving others barely hanging on to life?

Some might call it fate. Others, the will of God. That may be. But stroke patients and their families may be too quick to claim either one. "I often find that deep down inside, people who've suffered a terrible illness feel guilty that their behavior has caused the problem to happen," suggests Dr. John Corry, a chaplain who ministers to mostly black patients and families at Meharry Medical College's Hubbard Hospital in Nashville, Tennessee. "And so they feel God is punishing them for their mistakes. My approach is to help them see that God is compassionate and forgiving, that He allows things to happen, but He doesn't cause them." That helps people feel less guilty, and undoubtedly more eager to safeguard their health in the future.

After all, we may not understand our fate. But God certainly doesn't want us to neglect ourselves. Within our limited human understanding, if we know anything about illness and disease, it's that each of us can play a very real role in determining our health.

Medical School in Rochester, Minnesota. "Prevention of cerebrovascular disease provides not only the ideal, but also the only realistic approach to management."

If you don't know whether you or a loved one may be at high risk of having a stroke, it's easy to find out. In Chapter 2, we mentioned the factors that increase a person's risk for stroke—high blood pressure, older age, heart disease, family history of stroke, sickle cell anemia, and so forth. A doctor's examination, which should include a thorough medical history, can reveal how many of these risk factors are present, and how severe they are.

Let's assume you discover that you are indeed a high-risk candidate. You are a black man who has hypertension and you've already suffered a temporary ischemic attack. Or you're a black woman who smokes and uses oral contraceptives, and your doctor says you're in the early stages of heart disease. What are your options? Let's start our exploration of the options for African-Americans at risk by taking a close look at the principal cause of stroke in blacks: hypertension.

## OPTIONS FOR HYPERTENSION

By far the most dangerous and insidious risk factor for African-Americans is hypertension. It's dangerous because it can lead directly to a deadly cerebral hemorrhage or any number of other serious medical complications, from atherosclerosis to kidney failure. It's insidious because it causes no pain, so unless we keep track of our blood pressure and take steps to control it, we usually don't realize we're in trouble until it's too late.

Sadly, our track record for controlling hypertension leaves a lot to be desired. Hypertension in blacks is undiagnosed, untreated, and inadequately controlled for longer periods of time than for whites. "Only 50 percent of the black people who have high blood pressure are controlling it," says Dr. Edward Cooper, a pioneer in treating and preventing strokes in blacks, who wants to see better motivation and compliance push that figure to at least 75 percent. Compared to other groups, black men—the group with more high blood pressure than anyone else—have the worst record of controlling their hypertension.

Part of the problem, especially for blacks who are poor, is barriers in the medical care system: inconvenient clinic locations and hours of operation, long waiting times, and poor access to information about high blood pressure. Outside of the health care system, another piece of the problem stems from a social context that is hostile to African-Americans. Racism, unemployment, undereducation—these factors not only contribute to illness but often prevent us, either directly or indirectly, from getting the medical care that we need.

The cost of medication can be a real barrier to treating high blood pressure. Ironically, persons who are poor are more likely than others to have severely high blood pressure, which calls for higher doses of medicine—and more money. Many states refuse to provide Medicaid or Medicare coverage for managing hypertension. Dr. Neil Shulman of Emory University thinks that's a crime. "It just no longer makes sense for someone with high blood pressure and $8,000 in gross income to have to spend about $1,000—one-eighth of their gross income—for drugs to treat their disease."

But to be fair, part of the problem is our own behavior. We don't visit the doctor as often as we should. And when we do, we don't always follow the doctor's orders to take our medicine.

What kinds of medicine are we talking about? Several different types of drugs help alleviate high blood pressure. Doctors usually try them in stages—an approach that's sometimes referred to as "stepped care." The first line of defense is a *diuretic*. Diuretics cause fluids to leave the body through the urine. Relieving the body of some fluids is like easing air out of a balloon—it reduces the pressure inside the bloodstream.

In 20 to 40 percent of patients, including blacks, with mild or moderate hypertension, a diuretic is all it takes to lower blood pressure into the normal range.

If a patient needs stronger medicine, doctors often prescribe a so-called *sympathetic depressant* drug. "Sympathetic" isn't an attitude; it refers to a part of our nervous system. The sympathetic nervous system stimulates cells and organs, including the heart. When we climb stairs or get nervous before delivering a speech, it's the sympathetic nervous system that quickens our heartbeat, dries our mouth, opens our lungs, and slows down digestion. Sympathetic depressant medicines put a damper on these and other activities, and by slowing down the heart, helping the heart pump less blood with each beat, and relaxing the blood vessels, the medicines lower blood pressure. Beta blockers are one of the better known medicines in this group. Up to 80 percent of all cases of mild to moderate hypertension can be controlled by using the two-pronged combination of a diuretic and sympathetic depressant.

The third step, if necessary, is to add a *vasodilator.* This relaxes the blood vessels so that the fluids in the bloodstream are contained under less pressure.

A fourth option is to use a second sympathetic depressant.

These medicines work. One Veterans Administration study found that antihypertension medication reduced the risk of stroke and other complications of high blood pressure from 40 percent to a mere 3 percent. A larger study of nearly 460,000 middle-aged people from around the world found that after two to three years of taking antihypertension medicine, even a moderate 5-millimeter drop in diastolic blood pressure reduced the average person's risk of stroke by 40 percent. "We've known that a little bit of blood-pressure reduction goes a long way in reducing deaths from stroke," says Dr. Edward J. Roccella of the National High Blood Pressure Education Program. "But when you pool all the data like this, the magnitude is greater than we thought."

And antihypertension medicine works just as well in blacks as in whites. In fact, it may work even better. The Hypertension Detection and Follow-up Program, a five-year study by the National Institutes of Health, found that when white patients used antihypertension medicine in a strict stepped-care regimen, their death rate was 10 percent lower than white patients who merely continued to see their regular doctors for routine care. But for black patients in the same stepped-care program, the death rate plummeted to 22 percent below that of blacks who continued to get routine medical care elsewhere. Although many antihypertension drugs are effective in black patients, diuretics and vasodilators called calcium-entry blockers are particularly valuable.

But whether or not these medicines are actually effective depends on the person who is taking them—or *not* taking them, as the case may be. Unfortunately, when it comes to taking antihypertension medicine as prescribed, African-Americans don't always have the best track record. Many patients find that the medicine makes them sleepy or impotent, or gives them a dry mouth. These side effects are particularly pronounced in blacks because we are disproportionately overweight, and people who are overweight must take larger doses of medicine. Faced with these side effects, many black patients simply stop taking the medicine. They feel much better—until they have a stroke. This may be one reason that the southeastern states, with their high rates of African-American obesity and hypertension, are the nation's so-called Stroke Belt.

"If you have side effects, you should not stop taking your drugs," advises Dr. Edward J. Rocella, coordinator of the National High Blood Pressure Institute. "You should go back to your physician. He [or she] can adjust the medication." Changing the dose of the medicine or switching to another medication altogether can greatly relieve the side effects while continuing to reduce the hypertension.

Changing medications can also save money. A month's supply of a calcium-entry blocker can cost $60—well beyond the range of African-Americans who may be unemployed, underemployed, or living on a fixed income. But the same month's worth of a diuretic may run only $12. Sometimes there are no alternatives to expensive medicines. But in many cases, a thoughtful doctor can help bring hypertension control within a patient's budget.

Antihypertension medicine can be valuable for older persons. That's a dramatic departure from conventional wisdom. Not too long ago, doctors were resigned to the inevitable—that as people grew older, hypertension and strokes were an unavoidable one-two punch. Physicians knew that the stiffening of the arteries that comes with old age causes blood vessels to lose their elasticity, which means that the normally flexible blood-vessel wall can't act as a shock absorber for each heartbeat. The resulting rise in systolic (heart-pumping) blood pressure eventually causes a hemorrhage or ischemia. Physicians were reluctant to prescribe antihypertension medicine to their elderly patients for fear that the side effects would outweigh any benefits. They also had no proof that the medicines were effective in this age group.

But in 1991 came an electrifying study that may revolutionize how doctors approach stroke prevention in the elderly—and may especially benefit the elderly poor. The study tracked nearly five thousand elderly patients—20 percent of them persons of color—through a two-step program. Patients started the first step with low doses of chlorthalidone, a common diuretic. If necessary, some moved on to low doses of a beta blocker called atenolol. Because of the low doses, only 13 percent of the participants had to quit the study because of side effects. Best of all, this low-cost drug therapy, averaging about ten cents to twenty-five cents a day, slashed the risk of stroke by a full 36 percent. "This new finding is absolutely extraordinary," one of the researchers told *Science News* magazine. "It's one of the most exciting trials we've ever been involved in."

It's good news not only for people who are elderly today, but for the many baby boomers who will be at risk of stroke in record numbers in the early twenty-first century. Already researchers are concerned that although fewer people are dying of stroke these days, more people are having strokes. The fear is that the trend will get even worse as the average age of the population increases.

Medication is one of the most effective ways to control high blood pressure, particularly in severe cases. But there are other methods, too—methods that involve no medicine at all. In fact, for people with slight or moderate hypertension, these strategies often bring blood pressure neatly under control without ever having to take a single pill. Even for patients who have severe hypertension, doctors often recommend a number of measures to help strengthen the impact of blood-pressure medication. These measures follow, along with goals to aim for.

**Slim down.**
*Your weight loss goal is 5 percent (or more) of your current weight.*

As a rule, overweight people have higher blood pressure than do people of normal weight. And the more overweight you are, the higher your blood pressure.* Obesity causes salt retention and it increases the amount of blood in your arteries. Excess body weight also stimulates the sympathetic nervous system, causing our hearts to beat faster and our arteries to squeeze. As a person's weight increases, these triggers for hypertension become more and more severe. But miraculously, the reverse is true as well. "With weight reduction, all of these abnormalities disappear," says Dr. Timothy Caris, a hypertension expert and associate dean at the Medical School of the University of Texas Health Science Center.

And there's more good news: To reap your reward, you don't have to slim down to what you weighed in high school. High blood pressure often starts to improve when you lose as little as 5 percent of your body weight. That's as little as eight pounds for a one hundred fifty-pound person, or a ten-pound loss for a two hundred-pounder.

What's the best way to lose weight? Numerous studies of weight management verify that *diets don't work*. So spare yourself the expense of diet books and prepackaged formula plans. Just try to eat a little less and be a little more active. You must combine sound eating with more exercise; simply changing your eating habits doesn't work. Set a goal of losing weight at the ideal

---

*This rule isn't absolute. Some obese people have normal blood pressure.

rate: one to two pounds a month. That way, you will lose twelve to twenty-four pounds a year without being on a diet.

What do you get for your efforts? Quite a bit. On average, losing twenty-five pounds causes a drop of twenty-one points in systolic blood pressure and thirteen points in diastolic blood pressure. So by losing twenty-five pounds, a person with moderate hypertension* (blood pressure of 160/105, for example) could end up with only mild hypertension (blood pressure of 139/92). And a person with mild hypertension (blood pressure 150/90) could bring their blood pressure down to normal (129/77).

**Cut down on sodium.**
*Your sodium goal is 2,000 milligrams a day.*

You've seen it on television. You've read it on food labels. You may have even heard it from your doctor: virtually the only good thing about salt is how it tastes. Excess sodium is one of the chief causes of hypertension, and people who eat too much sodium soon run into problems. In Japan, a nation known for its salty cuisine, the stroke rate is the highest in the world.

Earlier, we touched on why too much sodium is bad news for our cardiovascular systems. Sodium causes our bodies to retain fluids that collect, among other places, inside our arteries and veins. The more fluids, the

---

*Doctors classify hypertension by the diastolic number, the lower of the two blood pressure numbers. (For blood pressure of 140/85, the diastolic number is 85.) Diastolic pressure is a measure of the blood pressure when the heart is at rest.

| Mild hypertension | 90–104 |
| Moderate hypertension | 105–114 |
| Severe hypertension | Over 115 |

## Six Tips for Losing Weight

1. Be gradual and realistic. If you didn't put on forty pounds in two months, why expect yourself to remove it in such a short time?

2. Remove calories that you won't miss. Skip the sugar in soft drinks (drink sugar-free soft drinks if you must) and cut down on the fat that you use to prepare foods. This change will both eliminate calories immediately and help your taste buds begin to enjoy foods without sugar and fat.

3. Teach yourself to be satisfied with one serving of the foods you have in front of you. How often have you eaten to the point of discomfort or pain? The only part of you that was happy was your tongue, where the taste buds are. Eating too much isn't inevitable; it's only a bad habit, not an addiction.

4. Feed your body, not your nerves. Try not to eat when you have the fidgets or are upset. If you must eat and you're anxious, try a warm liquid, such as soup or tea, instead of dessert or leftovers.

5. Be determined but flexible. Allow yourself special occasions and setbacks. Feel victorious that you have taken charge of your eating style and your weight.

6. Keep track of what you eat by keeping a daily log. The mere words staring back at you from a small pad can help you make better choices in the future.

higher a person's blood pressure. Our bodies need a bit of sodium to make sure that we retain a crucial amount of fluids. (On a sodium-free diet, we would become dehydrated.) But most Americans consume twenty to thirty times more sodium than their bodies need. And it shows—in our high rates of kidney disease, heart disease, and of course, stroke— diseases that are especially prevalent in the black community.

How much sodium is too much? Experts say we should hold the line at around 2,000 milligrams (mg) of sodium a day—about two teaspoons of salt. Most of us eat 4,000 to 6,000 milligrams per day. What many people don't realize is that much of the sodium we eat sneaks into our food without our knowing it. In fact, two-thirds of the sodium that we eat comes from processed foods. Processed meats, canned vegetables, salad dressings, and a number of other prepared foods are extremely salty. A Big Mac, medium fries, and chocolate shake at McDonald's delivers 1,280 milligrams of sodium. That's over half your daily allotment of sodium—without your ever lifting the salt shaker.

On the other hand, unprocessed foods such as fruits, vegetables, rice, vegetable oils, and fresh meats are remarkably low in sodium—usually less than 30 milligrams per serving. Appendix C gives the sodium content of common foods.

**Eat more potassium.**
*Your potassium goal is 3,500 milligrams a day.*

Sodium may be the most important dietary contribution to hypertension. But there are other dietary factors to keep in mind, too. For example, potassium is an important factor in high blood pressure. You may have heard doctors advise hypertensive patients to eat plenty of potassium-rich foods. The reason is that potassium and sodium help balance each other out. Our body's cells are surrounded by membranes that control the nutrients that flow in and the waste products that flow out. Once sodium makes its way into a cell, it begins to attract water—so much so that too much sodium can make a cell swell to the point of rupturing. How does it handle the excess? With a sodium "pump"—a chemical shuttle system that literally transports the extra sodium molecules safely across the cell membrane and out of the body via the kidneys. But the shuttle needs potassium to work. For every molecule of sodium that leaves the cell, a molecule of potassium enters. That's why doctors often recommend that hypertensive patients increase their potassium intake as they decrease their sodium intake. That's valuable advice for blacks, because the African-American diet is often very low in potassium.

Just as it doesn't take much of the wrong kind of food to send your sodium intake over the edge, it doesn't take much of the right kind to boost your potassium. Just one extra serving of fresh fruit or vegetables each day—one baked potato, one banana, one helping of greens, or an eight-ounce glass of orange or grapefruit juice—adds enough potassium to cut your risk of stroke by a whopping 40 percent.

Here's a simple formula for making sure that you have enough daily potassium: Each day, eat no less than three fruits or vegetables, and three times a week, eat a potato that's been cooked in the skin. You can be sure that you are eating a healthful amount of potassium if you fill half of your place at each meal with vegetables or fruits.

As fruits and vegetables are processed by food manufacturers, whether by canning, freezing, or dehydrating, their sodium content shoots up and their potassium content falls through the floor. So enjoy lots of fruits and vegetables, and choose those that are processed as little as possible. Appendix C lists the potassium content of common foods.

One final note: Potassium is good for you, but don't use a salt substitute containing potassium chloride without consulting your doctor. If you're taking certain medications, additional potassium may be unhealthy.

## Ways to Lick the Sodium Habit

- Do you use salt in cooking? If so, you can eliminate as much as 5,000 milligrams of sodium a day by using herb blends instead. Try emptying your salt shaker and filling it with a blend such as this:

### All-Purpose Spice Blend

5 t onion powder
2 ½ t garlic powder
2 ½ t paprika
2 ½ t powdered mustard
1 ¼ t thyme leaves
½ t ground white pepper
¼ t celery seed

Combine all ingredients and spoon into a shaker. Makes about one-third cup. Less than 1 milligram of sodium per teaspoon. (Courtesy of the American Spice Trade Association.)

Try tartness as a flavor zing. Vinegar, lemon or lime juice, or a sprinkle of grated citrus rind gives foods a wonderful kick. Boost your favorite barbeque or poultry flavors with more herbs. Here are some ideas:

| | |
|---|---|
| Fish herbs: | basil, bay leaf, lemon, thyme, parsley, tarragon, dill, garlic |
| Poultry herbs: | marjoram, sage |
| Salad herbs: | basil, parsley, tarragon |
| Tomato sauce herbs: | basil, bay leaf, marjoram, oregano, parsley, celery leaves |
| Vegetable herbs: | basil, chives, dill, tarragon, marjoram, mint, parsley, pepper, thyme |
| Barbeque blend: | cumin, garlic, hot pepper, oregano, chili powder |

- Do you eat out frequently? If so, expand your menu options. Choose fresh meat (e.g., turkey, roast beef, chicken) instead of salty cold cuts and cheeses. Lettuce and tomato are fine, but cut down on sodium-rich mustard, mayonnaise, and pickles. Salads without dressing or pickled vegetables are good choices. Foods made to order (such as baked potatoes, steamed vegetables, and broiled meats) can help you stay within your 2,000-milligram daily limit for sodium. Just ask that salt and soy sauce be omitted from your order.

(Adapted from *FDA Consumer,* April 1984)

**Load up on calcium.**
*Your calcium goal is 1,000 milligrams a day.*

Calcium helps the body maintain a healthy balance of minerals and fluids. The calcium in low-fat milk, yogurt, and cheese is easy for our bodies to absorb. So is the calcium in such traditional southern favorites as buttermilk and clabber (sour curdled milk). But as many as seven out of ten African-Americans cannot tolerate milk because they can't digest lactose, the sugar in milk. If you feel gas and cramping after you drink milk, look for low-lactose milk in your grocery store. You can also buy *lactase,* the enzyme that breaks down milk sugar to make it easier to digest, as tablets or drops in drugstores. If you're not a milk drinker, leafy vegetables (except for spinach) and canned fish (*with* the bones) are great sources of calcium. See Appendix C for others.

**Eat more magnesium.**
*Your magnesium goal is 300 to 350 milligrams a day.*

Magnesium helps regulate our blood pressure by controlling how our arteries squeeze. Appendix C gives good sources of magnesium.

**Fill up on fiber.**
*Your fiber goal is 30 grams a day.*

Fiber is the part of plants that people can't digest. It's the stuff that makes beans, vegetables, nuts, fruits, and grains (rice, wheat, corn, etc.) stringy, woody, or jellylike. The only way to get more fiber in your diet is to eat more foods that come from plants. Eat as much of the whole food as possible. That means eating the skin of an apple or potato instead of peeling it. You can also eat whole-wheat bread and cereal and brown rice instead of their refined (or white) counterparts. Appendix C lists the fiber content of many foods.

Fiber does more than lower your blood pressure. It also lowers your cholesterol levels. There are two types of fiber: water-insoluble (which is stringy or woody) and water-soluble (which is gummy or jellylike). Water-soluble fiber lowers blood cholesterol in a small but significant way. Here are some of the foods that contain water-soluble fiber:

| Kind of Soluble Fiber | Sources |
| --- | --- |
| gum | beans and peas, oat bran, seed, seaweed |
| pectin | apples, citrus fruits, berries, grapes |
| mucilage | seeds, okra |

Try to have at least three generous servings a day of a food that's high in soluble fiber. For example, you might build a menu around a large bowl of oatmeal for breakfast, a large apple with lunch, and a large bowl of bean soup or chili for dinner. Scientists don't know how dietary fiber helps lower blood pressure; one possibility is that fiber helps to signal the kidneys to retain less sodium.

**Cut down on alcohol.**
*Your goal is no alcohol. This is extremely important if you are pregnant.*

There's not much question that drinking causes high blood pressure. Doctors tell us that excess alcohol is one of the most important risk factors for hypertension. If you have more than a drink or two a day, chances are your cardiovascular system is paying the price.

Hypertension experts say that drinkers should hold the line at two ounces of alcohol per day. That's the equivalent of one twelve-ounce beer, eight ounces of wine, or as little as two ounces of spirits.

Alcohol is a dangerous, insidious drug in every community, but especially so in the African-American community. For black people, extraordinary stresses are the stuff of ordinary life. To help cope, African-Americans frequently turn to alcohol—a deadly decision that's encouraged by the presence of massive liquor-industry advertising encouraging blacks to drink. Fortunately, alcoholism is not inevitable; people with drinking problems can get help to learn how to manage their lives without resorting to alcohol. For help, see Appendix B.

**Kick the nicotine habit.**
*Your goal is no smoking.*

The deadliest form of high blood pressure is a condition called malignant hypertension. Once it starts, it progresses quickly, often ending in a life-threatening stroke or other complication. Smokers are much more likely to develop malignant hypertension than are people who don't smoke. Among other things, the nicotine in tobacco smoke is a stimulant that quickens the heartbeat and tightens a person's blood vessels. If you smoke, cutting down on tobacco or cutting it out of your life entirely will do your cardiovascular system— not to mention your lungs—a world of good.

Cigarette smoking can be among the most difficult addictions to break, and African-Americans are at special risk. Black people smoke more often than do whites and tend to favor menthol cigarettes. The menthol acts as a mild anesthetic, which allows smokers to inhale deeper, thereby bringing noxious gases and toxic chemicals farther into the lungs. Peer pressure often encourages adolescents to begin a lifetime of smoking at an early age, and cigarette manufacturers add their persuasive voices by persistently targeting the black community with the implied message that smokers get more enjoyment from life. A decade ago, former U.S. Health and Human Services Secretary Dr. Louis Sullivan drew national attention to the marketing of tobacco to blacks—a community already disproportionately beset by disease—when he criticized the R.J. Reynolds Company for launching Uptown cigarettes in an unabashed attempt to capture the black smokers' market. R.J. Reynolds withdrew the product.

Despite these pressures, more and more smokers can and do successfully give up cigarettes every day. There are even self-help aids for black smokers. See Appendix B for details.

### Work up a little sweat.*
*Your goal is vigorous exercise three times a week.*

You can be eighty or eighteen, black or white—exercise does wonders for hypertension. A regular program of energetic, heart-pumping activity—brisk walking, jogging, swimming, cycling—can cause resting (diastolic) blood pressure to drop anywhere from five to fifteen points. For African-Americans, regular exercise also seems to lower nighttime blood pressure, which is often elevated compared to whites—a fact that may help explain why blacks have higher overall blood pressure.

---

*Note: Hypertension places a person at risk of stroke, heart disease, and other serious complications, so anyone with hypertension should consult a physician before starting an exercise program.

To benefit your heart and blood vessels, the exercise must satisfy three ground rules: (1) you have to exercise moderately vigorously (2) twenty to thirty minutes per session (3) at least three times a week. If you're unaccustomed to this sort of regimen, start with modest goals. As your body begins to respond by slowly easing back into shape, the goals can be modified.

Exercise is like a computer: over the years, it becomes user-friendly. Twenty or thirty years ago, exercising meant pulling on bulky sweatpants and heavy sneakers and dutifully enduring a lonely chore. Today, lightweight, fashionable clothing and shoes make exercising more enjoyable. Walkman radios and tape players provide pleasant distractions. Exercising no longer means pushing yourself to the point of exhaustion. "We spend time debunking some common myths, such as the coaches' rule of 'No Pain, No Gain,'" explains Dr. Patricia Dubbert, whose Jackson, Mississippi, Veterans Administration Center runs an extensive exercise program for its middle-aged and elderly clients. "Pain-free, low levels of aerobic exercise are essentially equivalent in the overall cardiovascular training effects to very high levels."

Best of all, we have become a nation of exercisers, and it's easy now to find friends, family members, fellow workers, and neighborhood acquaintances to exercise with. (Studies show that people who exercise with someone else are twice as likely as people who exercise alone to stick with an exercise program.) In many areas of the country, organized exercise programs seem to have cropped up on nearly every street corner. Hospitals, YMCAs and YWCAs, local health departments, universities, and many corporations have fitness programs that help provide the motivation and support people need to start a good exercise program and stick with it.

All of this is good news, indeed, because exercise does a lot more than just lower your blood pressure. For one thing, it burns off calories. Regular vigorous exercise not only eats up calories during the exercise session, but also speeds up the body's metabolism, so that the body burns more calories even between sessions. That's why exercise is a valuable part of any weight-loss program.

Regular exercise also raises the level of HDL (high density lipoprotein), a beneficial cholesterol that is known to reduce the risk of heart disease.

Finally, exercise is a marvelous tool for emotional health. It reduces anxiety, relieves depression, and makes a person feel relaxed and tranquil. Some psychologists believe that exercise also delivers something that African-Americans sometimes have in short supply: a feeling of control. Exercisers know that they are taking positive steps to improve their well-being, and the sense of accomplishment and mastery that they gain is often palpable. "I actually see a physical change in my clients," New York psychologist Francesca Casciaro told the *New York Times*. "The relief of stress in the body and the face is immediately evident."

### Chill out.
Black Americans get it from all sides. We have a tougher time landing a job, then we have to fight harder to keep it. We're doubted in the classroom and locked out of the boardroom. We live in the dirtiest neighborhoods, get the worst health care, and hold the least political power. As the saying goes, when America sneezes, we get pneumonia.

In the midst of these and other high-pressure stresses, nobody claims that relaxing is easy. But if you can figure out ways to beat stress, it can not only make life more livable, but reduce your blood pressure as well.

The theory behind stress management as a form of hypertension control is simple. When our blood pressure increases, it's usually because our nervous system is aroused. Maybe someone has made us angry or irritable, or we're hard-driving and competitive on the job, or we're rushing too fast to do too many things. If nervous system arousal hikes up blood pressure, it makes sense that learning to control that arousal can decrease your blood pressure.

Stress management means different things to different people. To some, it means psychotherapy or biofeedback. Others may manage stress by taking a class in time management or assertiveness training. One of the more popular forms of stress management is relaxation therapy, a concept that can mean meditation or something called progressive muscle relaxation, which involves flexing and relaxing all of the major muscle groups in the body.

Regardless of the technique, relaxation therapy works. When hypertensive patients take time to practice relaxation therapy on a regular basis, their diastolic blood pressure can fall as many as twenty to thirty points or more.

## OPTIONS FOR PREVENTING HEART DISEASE

After hypertension, heart disease ranks high on the list of important risk factors for stroke. Fortunately for African-Americans, it also ranks high on the list of diseases that we can prevent. The principal strategy with heart disease is keeping close tabs on our fat and cholesterol intake.

### Eat less fat.
*Your goal is 50 to 60 grams per day.*

There's "bad fat" and there's "not-so-bad fat." Hard fat—any fat from a four-legged animal, as well as the fat from hydrogenated oils and palm kernel oils—is the worst. This is also called *saturated fat,* and it's the kind of fat that's prone to clog our arteries and lead to heart attacks and stroke. *Monounsaturated* and *polyunsaturated* fats are less damaging to the body. So it's best to focus on eliminating saturated fats from our diets first. It's not that difficult, really: simply reduce your intake of red meat to five ounces a day or less, don't use animal fats (lard, butter, bacon grease, etc.) in cooking, and use liquid or soft vegetable fats when you cook. Remember that most of us eat too much fat in general, so fats of all kinds should be trimmed from our diets. If you shoot for about 50 to 60 grams of fat per day, with no more than 10 percent of the total comprising saturated fat, you'll be eating in the range that nutritionists advise. Appendix C describes sources of various fats.

### Cut the cholesterol.
*Your goal is less than 300 milligrams a day.*

If you've met your goals for fat, you've already mastered your goal for cholesterol! Here's why: Cholesterol is made only by the liver. That means that cholesterol will only—and always—be in foods that either come from animals (such as beef, chicken, pork, and fish) or have ingredients that come from animals (such as eggs,* whole milk, and cheese). Thus, to limit your cholesterol intake, you need only put a lid on how much "animal foods" you eat, limiting "flesh" to five ounces a day, selecting only skimmed-milk dairy products, and replacing all animal fats in cooking with vegetable fats. In so doing, you'll easily fall under 300 milligrams of cholesterol a day.

In addition to limiting our fat and cholesterol intake, there are other ways to prevent heart disease. Getting regular exercise and giving up cigarettes are two of the most important ways to build a strong, healthy heart and maintain a youthful cardiovascular system.

## ONE GOOD HABIT, MANY BENEFITS

Many of our daily transactions are simple one-to-one exchanges. A waiter serves us; we tip him. A friend does us a favor; we reciprocate. But when people take care of their health, they often discover that one healthful habit brings not one benefit but lots of them. This pleasant revelation makes sense, when you think of it. After all, bad habits hurt the body in more than one way, too.

The chance to get lots of "bang for the buck" is great news for Africans-Americans at risk of stroke. It means that the measures you take to reduce your stroke risk can pay off lots of other ways.

---

*Egg substitutes and other fat-free and cholesterol-free products that you find in grocery stores can be eaten liberally.

Take weight loss, for example. By now, you know that controlling your weight helps guard against hypertension and reduce your chances of a stroke. But obesity is a major risk factor in a number of other serious health disorders, including heart disease and diabetes. So people who keep their weight within healthy limits are helping themselves avoid at least three diseases.

Two other good dietary habits—cutting back on sodium and taking in plenty of potassium—bring multiple payoffs, too. One good way to reduce your sodium intake is to go easy on fast food, which is notoriously salty. But too many burgers and fried chicken and deep-fried fish filets at America's fast-food franchises are also loaded with fat and cholesterol. Over time, too much fat can lead to diabetes or breast or colon cancer. It can also turn a healthy, flexible artery into a stiffened, fat-clogged accident waiting to happen. So replacing some of the fast food in your diet with more healthful alternatives can do a world of good *and* cut your stroke risk, too.

Likewise, potassium is abundant in fruit and vegetables, which are high in dietary fiber. A healthy intake of fiber can guard against constipation, diverticulosis, and colon cancer.

The list goes on. Giving up smoking is a superb way to ward off lung cancer as well as heart disease and stroke. Regular exercise tones muscles, increases joint flexibility, and relieves stress. Drinking alcohol in moderation, if at all, helps avoid birth defects, brain damage, cirrhosis of the liver, and cancers of the throat and mouth.

## OTHER PREVENTIVE MEASURES

Controlling high blood pressure and preventing heart disease are excellent ways to prevent strokes, but they aren't the only tool in the medical arsenal. For persons who are beginning to show warning signs of an impending stroke, drug therapy can often arrest the damage and sometimes even reverse it. In more extreme cases where medicines won't work, surgery can be a very effective way to head off a stroke before it erupts.

Finally, there's a way of preventing stroke that doesn't involve medicine or surgery, and it doesn't cost a cent. It may very well surprise you. But that's jumping ahead. So let's examine each of these options in more detail.

### Blood Thinners

Blood has a natural tendency to clot. It's a godsend that helps us heal when we are injured. Unfortunately, clots are responsible for a large number of strokes, too. Blood thinners come to the rescue by preventing clots from forming. And if you stop the clot, you prevent the stroke.

Coumadin, the most widely used blood thinner, is also known by the generic name "warfarin." Doctors often prescribe warfarin for a common heart disorder called *atrial fibrillation* (ay´-tree-ul fib-ri-lay´shun), in which nerve messages that coordinate the heartbeat become confused, causing the upper chambers of the heart (the atria) to quiver instead of pump. When that happens, some of the blood that normally leaves the heart in smooth, steady pulses can pool inside the heart chambers, where it begins to clot. Of course, if the clot then leaves the heart and travels to the brain, it can cause a stroke. Atrial fibrillation, which affects one million elderly Americans, causes about seventy-five thousand strokes each year—15 percent of the national total. Low doses of warfarin can cut the risk of stroke by an impressive 70 percent.

Warfarin has two disadvantages—side effects and cost. Too much of the drug can overthin the blood and actually cause bleeding. Doctors guard against this by prescribing low doses, thereby keeping the risk of serious complications to around 1 percent. But the potential for bleeding means that patients who take warfarin need to have their blood tested, once a week at first, then once every month or so. The combination of the testing and the medicine itself generally runs around $500 per year.

There's a much more affordable blood thinner on the market, and it's probably already in your medicine cabinet. Ordinary aspirin, the bane of headaches and fever, can prevent strokes, and for as little as two or three cents a day. In fact, aspirin is now standard therapy after a TIA or other stroke. "It's safe, inexpensive, and potentially effective. What could be better?" asks Dr. Robert Hart, who studies aspirin and stroke at the University of Texas Health Science Center in San Antonio.

Like all medicines, aspirin should be taken only under a doctor's care. The reason is that aspirin, like warfarin, does such a good job preventing blood from clotting that it can cause bleeding. In a worst-case scenario, aspirin taken to prevent an ischemic stroke (which is caused by a blood clot) can cause a hemorrhagic stroke (which is caused by bleeding). That's why the director of the National Heart, Lung, and Blood Institute in Bethesda was cautious when he announced new findings on the value of aspirin. "The last thing I want to see is everybody rush to the drug store and take aspirin every day," warned Dr. Claude Lenfant.

But when used properly, blood thinners—whether we're talking about warfarin or aspirin—work. And they work dramatically well. Consider what happened as aspirin and warfarin were being tested in a group of patients with atrial fibrillation. When scientists test a drug, they usually divide volunteers into two groups. One group gets the real drug; the other gets an identical placebo, or sugar pill. When the first results of the test arrived, the volunteers who took sugar pills had had so many more strokes than those who took the real medicine that the researchers did something virtually unheard of: they abruptly stopped the study in midstream, revealed who was taking placebos, and started giving everyone blood thinners.

If every American with atrial fibrillation took one of these two medicines, it would prevent an estimated one hundred to one hundred fifty strokes each *day*.

### Ultrasound

"It could prevent hundreds of strokes each year," predicts Dr. Robert Adams of the Medical College of Georgia. Dr. Adams is proud of a device he has developed to identify sickle cell anemia patients who are at risk of stroke. Sickle cell anemia, you'll recall, elongates a person's red blood cells, causing them to accumulate inside the patient's blood vessels instead of flowing through unimpeded. The minute blood vessels of the brain are especially vulnerable. One in every four hundred black infants is born with the disease. And before they reach adulthood, as many as 7 percent of these babies have strokes serious enough to cause paralysis. Doctors don't know why some sickle cell children and not others develop blocked arteries, and before Dr. Adams came along, they had no way of predicting who would fall victim to a stroke. But with ultrasound technology, African-American children and their families have a new tool in the battle against an infamous genetic disorder.

Dr. Adams realized that when blood passes through a narrowed region in an artery, it speeds up. By using sound waves to measure the speed of blood in the brain's arteries, the ultrasound machine spots a sign of arterial narrowing that might one day cause a stroke. That can give doctors a chance to step in with preventive treatment, which might consist of giving the children periodic blood transfusions.

As a preventive tool for sickle cell patients, ultrasound is still in the testing stages. But early indications, based on work with several hundred at-risk black children in Georgia, are promising. The device is "certainly innovative," Dr. Joy Samuels-Reid of Howard University's Center for Sickle Cell Disease told the Associated Press when news of Dr. Adams's machine was announced in January 1991. "I see no reason why it shouldn't help."

### Estrogen

For seven years during the 1980s, nearly nine thousand female residents of Leisure World, a retirement community near Los Angeles, made a unique contribution to medicine. The women took part in a study to figure out whether estrogen, a female hormone, protects against stroke. The production of estrogen by

the ovaries declines when a woman enters menopause; hot flashes, cold sweats, depression, and other
uncomfortable symptoms of menopause are in fact
caused by this slowdown in hormone production.

At the University of Southern California, Dr. Annlia
Paganini-Hill realized that estrogen supplements reduce LDL cholesterol (the cholesterol that contributes to the fatty deposits in atherosclerosis). So she
prevailed on the women of Leisure World to help her
find some answers. Seven years later, the results were
in: Forty-three women who took placebos had a
stroke, compared to only twenty cases of stroke
among women who took estrogen. After years of spec-
ulation, it was the first solid indication that estrogen
supplements protect against stroke. Future studies will
undoubtedly clarify the value of the hormone.

Drug therapy always involves a trade-off, and if estrogen does in fact help women avoid a stroke, patients
will have to weigh this benefit against the risks of estrogen supplements, which are thought to include heart
disease and cancer of the breast and uterus.

### Surgery*

It's riskier than an exercise program. And at $5,000
to $10,000, it's a lot more expensive than watching
your sodium intake. But for persons who are on a colli-
sion course with a stroke and who can't be helped any
other way, surgery can reduce the risk dramatically.

---

*This section does not cover bypass surgery, in which a surgeon uses a
portion of a blood vessel to build a bridge around a blocked artery in
the brain. Bypass surgery has been performed since the late 1960s, and
it is known to have restored normal blood flow to the brain in some patients. However, doctors do not agree on the conditions that make a
patient suitable for a bypass, and we simply don't know as much about
the procedure as we do about carotid endarterectomy.

One of the signs of impending stroke is the buildup of fatty deposits in the bloodstream. These tend to collect in the neck where the carotid artery branches off into two smaller arteries. In 1954, surgeons decided to try to remove the fatty plaque by opening the artery and carefully stripping the plaque from the blood vessel wall. The idea was to prevent a slowly growing clot from one day obstructing the artery completely—and causing a stroke. By 1985, 107,000 of the operations—called a carotid endarterectomy—were being performed each year.

But by the mid-1980s, trouble began to brew. For one thing, doctors received new information on the risks of the operation. The chance of dying from complications after a carotid endarterectomy stood at about 3 percent. But for a person with clogged carotid arteries and no warning signs of a stroke, the chance of having a fatal stroke within a year's time was only 2 percent. In other words, operating was riskier than not operating. "These findings came as a tremendous shock to the surgical and medical community," one federal health policymaker told the *New York Times*. With risks that high, some doctors said, lots of patients would be better off avoiding surgery and using medication to reduce fatty arterial deposits.

What's more, there was no solid evidence that the operation did any good. One study found that for patients whose neck arteries were blocked 30 percent or less, the surgery did nothing to prevent a future stroke. By the end of the decade, carotid endarterectomies were losing popularity. "What is painfully obvious," one stroke expert wrote in the *New England Journal of Medicine*, "is that we still don't know which patients, with what lesions [fatty deposits], detected by which tests, should be treated, and with which therapies."

An answer came soon enough. In 1991, the news spread that for patients with severely narrowed carotid arteries, the surgery indeed worked—and worked better, in fact, than anyone had expected. Research at dozens of hospitals showed that patients whose neck arteries were so clogged that 70 to 99 percent of the blood could not flow through were prime candidates for the operation. In these patients, all of whom had recently suffered a TIA or other non-disabling stroke, surgery worked better than blood thinners. Of 659 high-risk patients who received warfarin or aspirin, 26 percent had strokes within two years. Only 9 percent of patients who went through surgery had later strokes. (Surgery was ineffective in patients whose neck arteries were not severely blocked.)

So for persons who are seriously ill—those who have already suffered one stroke and seem headed for another, for example—surgery may be a valuable option. Anyone contemplating this operation should remember that the surgery is still risky. In inexperienced hands, carotid endarterectomies can lead to serious complications, including death. If a piece of fatty material breaks off as the surgeon is trying to remove it and finds its way into the bloodstream, it can, ironically, cause a stroke.

Patients and family members can do much to minimize these risks. Remember first of all that decisions about this operation shouldn't be rushed. Doctors usually first find carotid narrowing by listening through a stethoscope for a bruit—the distinctive sound that blood makes when it flows past an obstruction. But the mere presence of a bruit does not mean that someone should have an operation. A doctor should take a thorough, detailed history to determine whether the clogging of the arteries is confined to the neck or is more widespread. Diagnostic tests, including an angiography and CT scan, are usually performed to find out how extensive the blockage is. (Remember, the surgery is only effective if a patient's arteries are severely blocked.) If the diagnostic exams show extensive blockage, the patient's medical condition should be carefully evaluated to see if he or she is a good candidate for surgery.

To minimize the risks of surgery, patients and their families should try to have the operation performed at a hospital that has experience with the procedure. It's good to ask how many years the operation has been performed at the hospital and the percentage of patients who have complications after surgery. To put these numbers in perspective, you can ask for the names of other facilities that perform carotid endarterectomies and pose the same questions to them. Then compare answers. (Studies show that at some community hospitals, the risk of the surgery causing a stroke is a sky-high 21 percent. At a good hospital, the overall rate of death or serious disease from a carotid endarterectomy should fall under 4 percent, according to Dr. Robert Ratcheson, chief of neurosurgery at the Case Western Reserve School of Medicine.)

Finally, not all surgeons at a given facility have the same degree of experience with a given procedure. It's okay to ask which surgeon has the best record and then ask that that doctor perform the operation or at least be present in the operating room. All of these steps—making sure a patient is evaluated carefully and that an operation is performed at a high-quality facility by experienced hands—will help minimize the risks of a carotid endarterectomy and help guarantee that the operation successfully prevents a stroke.

As for covering the high cost of the operation, one of the best options for African-Americans over age sixty-five is Medicare, which will pay for the surgery.

## Upbeat Disposition

What does mood have to do with strokes? Plenty, says Susan Everson of the California Department of Health. Everson followed over 6,000 California adults starting in 1965 when they averaged forty-three years old. At that time, they filled out a questionnaire that asked about symptoms of depression. Twenty-nine years later, one in twenty-five depressed people had experienced a stroke, compared with one in forty-four people who weren't depressed.

"Prolonged states of depressed mood have effects on the body," Duke University Medical Center psychologist John Barefoot told *USA Today* when the depression study was released in 1997. To be specific, depression alters the activity of platelets—blood cells responsible for clotting—in a way that makes stroke-triggering clots more prone to happen. People who are depressed may also be more stroke-prone because they have higher heart rates, experience more stress hormones, and are less willing to take their medications as prescribed.

You don't have to put on a happy face, especially if that's not your natural disposition. Just try to avoid placing yourself in situations where you may feel depressed. "People should be doing something about depression, even if it's just exercise that lifts the mood, or short-term therapy," says Barefoot.

## A PEP TALK

Talk with ten people who have been through a stroke, and chances are they will all tell you the same thing: they would have done anything to avoid it. What many people don't realize is just how much they could have done to prevent it. There's a great deal that we still don't know about stroke. We don't understand everything there is to know about why some people recover more fully than others. We don't know nearly as much about treating strokes as we do about preventing them. We don't have all the answers to how the brain heals, or when surgery is the best preventive option. (We'll talk more in the next chapter about how science is uncovering new answers to some of these age-old questions about stroke.)

But one thing we have a fairly good handle on is what causes strokes. We know that uncontrolled hypertension is an open invitation for a stroke. We know that heart disease stacks the deck against us a little more. We know that smoking cigarettes and drinking too much alcohol make things even worse. And we know that all of these conditions are particularly widespread in the black community, thereby placing us at special risk.

We also know that when you control these risk factors, you control your chances of having a stroke. In fact, stroke protection is just one of the many benefits. By exercising, kicking tobacco, watching your pressure, and so forth, stroke protection is just one of the many benefits that will come your way. You'll also protect yourself from hypertension, heart disease, lung cancer—and maybe even Alzheimer's disease. Researchers at the University of Kentucky have found

that TIAs may cause much of the memory loss and dementia that's associated with Alzheimer's. The logical
conclusion: keep the risk factors for stroke under control, and you may simultaneously prevent a frightening and poorly understood disorder that slowly eats
away at the minds of 4 million Americans.

Not every risk factor is controllable, of course. We
can't do much to change our age, or our gender, or
our family health history. But many of the important
risk factors are squarely within our power to change.
And that means strokes are preventable. What it takes
is a little information, a little motivation, and a little
dedication. Information, motivation, and dedication—think of these as the three ingredients you need
to do the right thing.

*Information* helps us know what to do. The more we
know the facts about stroke, the more we can plan a
healthful lifestyle, one that features a good diet, regular
exercise, no smoking, and moderate drinking (or none
at all). And don't forget regular visits with your doctor.
Lots of African-Americans don't realize they have hypertension, diabetes, and other serious diseases, because we see a doctor only when a health problem is so
severe that we simply cannot bear the discomfort any
longer. By this time, an illness is often in the advanced
stages, which means it is difficult to treat. What's more,
instead of being treated as outpatients, persons who
wait this long before seeking care sometimes have to be
admitted to a hospital, which invariably means much
higher costs. Regular checkups with your doctor can
spot small problems before they become big ones, and
can help control chronic conditions (such as hypertension and heart disease) before they get worse. How
often should you get a checkup? Your doctor can tell

you, based on your age, your family history, your lifestyle, and your overall health.

One last thing about information: we need to overcome our fear of it. Sometimes, black people apparently feel that the best way to insulate themselves from a harsh reality is not to acknowledge it. Have you ever heard a lively conversation about a mutual acquaintance suddenly turn to whispers when someone mentions the person's illness, particularly if the illness is serious? Have you ever realized that you know a lot about a relative, except the circumstances surrounding their illness or death? There's something about serious health matters that we often consider taboo. When it comes to news about disease or death, we don't want to hear about it, talk about it, or think about it. Maybe it's because for too many of us, the news is bad. We hear about Grandpa John's stroke on Wednesday and by the weekend he's passed away. Or we hear that by the time surgeons operated on Sister Emily, her cancer was too widespread to save her. We don't realize that Grandpa John and Sister Emily might have saved themselves by seeing a doctor early on. All we know is that the people closest to us were with us one day and gone the next. No wonder we're reluctant to confront our health head-on: we don't feel that we have control. Overcoming this reluctance is the first step in taking charge of our health. Once that hurdle is passed and we become receptive to information, the doors to good health begin to open.

*Motivation* is what keeps us going, even when we have to plunge in against the current. It's not always easy to do the right thing for our health. Sometimes the pressures of everyday living are so urgent that taking care of our health doesn't seem nearly as important as making sure our children are fed and clothed, bringing home enough money to cover all the bills, settling a dispute with a landlord, or tending to the needs of a spouse or partner. In the face of these sorts of daily stresses, it's easy to feel that you just don't have enough time to be healthy. But you might be surprised that *anyone* can take steps to ensure their health, and it doesn't necessarily take very much time. It doesn't take much time or energy to watch how much sodium we eat, or to make sure we have plenty of potassium-rich fruits and vegetables at the table. Eating a wholesome diet is an important part of keeping high blood pressure under control. Likewise, starting an exercise habit takes only an hour or two a week, but it pays off not only by helping to keep hypertension and heart disease in check but by keeping us limber, youthful-feeling, and better able to deal with those everyday stresses.

Some of us may find it easier to look after someone else's health than our own. In the African-American community, women have traditionally been the caretakers for their men, their children, and frequently their grandchildren. Women may focus so entirely on the needs of others that they neglect their own. If you are a caretaker, find a way to work your needs into the picture. The best way to provide for your loved ones is to stay healthy yourself. By practicing good health habits, you can also use your influence in your family and in your community to quietly set an example for others.

And finally, *dedication*. Dedication means having the diligence to take your hypertension medication day in and day out, even when you're tempted to skip it because you don't feel sick. Or to try to quit smoking one more time even though your past three attempts didn't last very long. Or to keep searching for an exercise program that's enjoyable and convenient when your life is already busy and you've never considered yourself very athletic in the first place.

Dedication is what it takes to stick with the program when it would be far easier to give up. African-Americans may run a higher risk of having a stroke, but when it comes to dedication, we have a clear advantage: if black people had given up in the face of adversity, we wouldn't be here today. We've known for generations that in the final analysis, the only people we can rely on to make sure we are healthy, in mind and body and spirit, are ourselves.

# CHAPTER 6

# New Hope, New Dreams

The brown-skinned man stood at the podium and surveyed his audience. He was the first African-American to hold his job, so in a sense everything he said set a precedent. But to black Americans, this day would be memorable for another reason. After discussing statistics about stroke and outlining promising new research, the black man would wrap up his speech with two stunning predictions: by the end of this decade, not only will doctors know how to protect the brain during acute strokes, but 80 percent of all strokes will be prevented from occurring in the first place.

Bold words, perhaps. But Dr. Louis Sullivan was speaking on good authority. Sullivan, the first black Secretary of the U.S. Department of Health and Human Services, knew that strokes are the nation's third most frequent killer. He knew that stroke patients, particularly the poor and people of color, can't always get affordable, quality health care. And still, Dr. Sullivan was convinced that the rate of disease and death from stroke would plummet within a very few years. What could have persuaded the secretary to make such a bold prediction?

## THE RESEARCH ASSAULT ON STROKE

Secretary Sullivan knew that there is a war on stroke. And he knew that scientists and doctors aren't the only ones who are winning. Stroke patients are, too.

Take tPA, for example. tPA stands for tissue plasminogen activator. It's a chemical that the body produces to dissolve blood clots once they have served their purpose (which is usually stopping the flow of blood from a wound). Once inside the bloodstream, tPA is active for only about ten minutes. This gives it an advantage over more long-lasting clot dissolvers such as warfarin, because it doesn't stick around long enough to cause bleeding. When researchers at the Burroughs Wellcome pharmaceutical firm gave tPA to patients soon after the onset of an ischemic stroke, the blood clots in one-third of the patients broke up partially or completely within an hour.

Now that scientists know tPA can help remove clots, the National Institutes of Health is studying the chemical's ability to help stroke patients function again. And they like what they're finding. In NIH-sponsored research on 624 stroke patients, those who received tPA were 30 percent or more likely to have minimal or no disabilities compared to those who received a placebo. "Yesterday, stroke was an untreatable disease," said one scientist. "Today, it is treatable."

A second approach to treating stroke is a class of medicines known as neuroprotectants. One of these, a medication called citicoline, works by, among other things, supplying the building blocks needed to repair damaged nerve cell membranes. In tests, stroke-damaged patients who received citicoline scored higher on learning and memory than did patients who received only a placebo.

Remedies like tPA and citicoline are valuable because not all of the brain damage from a stroke happens immediately. Individual neurons may begin to deteriorate within anywhere from a few minutes to many hours, depending on how much of their blood supply is blocked. There's not much that science can do for neurons at the center of the stroke-affected region, where the blood supply is severely restricted. But for adjacent areas of the brain that can still get part of their blood supply from other arteries, researchers are beginning to understand exactly what happens during the important time period after a stroke, so they can prevent endangered neurons from dying.

Part of the puzzle seems to be tied to a chain reaction called the "glutamate cascade." When neurons lose their blood supply, they start to send out huge amounts of a stimulant called glutamate. In the healthy brain, glutamate is a key messenger chemical that, among other things, helps the brain create long-term memory. But in a stroke-damaged brain, glutamate goes haywire, overexciting every other neuron within reach. It attaches to special bonding sites on nearby nerve cells, where it flings open the door for a fatal influx of calcium. The calcium quickly overwhelms neighboring neurons. In a dying act, each one pumps out more glutamate, which overexcites still other neurons. The chain reaction continues from cell to cell, leaving dead and dying neurons in its wake.

Stop this chain reaction, scientists promise, and you can halt the deterioration as a patient moves from the acute stage of stroke to the so-called completed stage, where brain damage is essentially complete. It's a little like trying to singlehandedly stop a wild team of runaway horses, but on a microscopic scale.

Dr. Raymond Swanson says he has one answer: never let the horses out of the barn. Swanson, a researcher at the University of California at San Francisco, may have a way to prevent stroke-damaged neurons from producing so much glutamate. If you can stop the glutamate cascade at the source, he says, there will be nothing to trigger the chain reaction.

Another strategy is preventing glutamate from reaching neighboring neurons. Several new drugs act on the receptor sites of these neurons, essentially denying the stimulant docking privileges. One such drug, dextromethorphan, is the active ingredient in certain cough medicines. Another, MK-801, is closely related to the street drug angel dust, and must be used with care. These so-called glutamate-receptor blockers show great promise. Experts predict that when the new medicines become widely available, they may eventually prevent brain damage in up to 80 percent of stroke patients.

But if you think glutamate-receptor blockers are impressive, Stanford University researcher Dr. Dennis Choi calls them "blunt axes" compared to elegant new drugs that disrupt the glutamate cascade once it gets under way. For example, in one step in the deadly cascade, a microscopic shuttle system carries a potentially toxic enzyme to a neuron's doorstep. Medicines called gangliosides put the brakes on the shuttle, stranding the enzyme at a safe distance from the neuron during the vulnerable hours that follow a stroke.

At another stage in the cascade, a dying neuron releases a swarm of special oxygen molecules that attack the delicate membrane surrounding neighboring neurons. Once that membrane starts to wither, the contents of the neuron literally start leaking out. Just as crucial, compounds residing outside the neuron's membrane—compounds like our old villain calcium—start to leak in. A drug called methylprednisolone seems to penetrate the cell membrane like a suit of armor, making it more resilient against the damaging effects of the oxygen.

At Columbia University, chemists are fashioning remarkable compounds patterned after—of all things—wasp venom. Egyptian digger wasps love to feast on honey bees, which they feed to their young. They manage this delicate feat by paralyzing the bees with a venom that blocks the bees' nerve messages. These messages are normally conveyed via—you guessed it—glutamate, the same chemical messenger that resides in the human brain. The venom clogs the bee's docking ports for glutamate, preventing the transmission of nerve messages that the bee's tiny muscles need to fight or fly away. The Columbia researchers hope that man-made venom substitutes will help them better understand how glutamate receptors work, thereby hastening the development of medicines that block the effects of glutamate.

Snakes are providing another of nature's contribution in the fight against stroke. Venom from the Malayan pit viper promotes bleeding; animals bitten by the snake bleed to death because their blood can't clot. But as we know from aspirin and warfarin, substances that cause bleeding are useful against blood clots. And in fact, that's why scientists are interested in viper venom. They think it may by a good way to dissolve blood clots in ischemic stroke patients.

If you can't dissolve a clot, what about flushing it out of a tight space? That's essentially what Dr. John G. Frazee and colleagues at the UCLA Medical Center are doing in a daring attempt to bypass a stroke patient's circulatory system. Blood usually flows through veins away from the brain. Dr. Frazee reverses this flow by pumping oxygen-rich blood from a patient's veins into the area of the brain where a clot is causing a stroke. There the veins give the brain an entirely fresh blood supply, and the clot either dissolves or is flushed away by the reverse-flowing blood. "The front door to the brain is blocked by a clot," the neurosurgeon told the Associated Press. "We decided to use the back door." In experimental tests, four of six patients who were treated soon after a stroke had virtually complete recovery.

What's better than messing with a blood clot at all? How about preventing it from forming in the first place? At the Scripps Research Foundation in La Jolla, California, Dr. Thomas Edgington is trying to unravel what makes blood clot. Edgington and his colleagues know that clotting is a multistage chemical reaction involving specialized blood cells and twenty-eight different proteins. The trick is to figure out the very first event that triggers the rest of the chain. The answer seems to center around tissue factor (TF), a protein that somehow starts the formation of arterial plaque. By inhibiting TF, Edgington and others hope to help people at risk—TIA patients, for example—avoid a full-blown stroke.

The list of experimental treatments for strokes is long and varied. Many experimental drugs are being tested on humans; more are becoming available to stroke patients each year. In the past decade or two, the sheer amount of exciting new information on preventing stroke damage has been unprecedented. "At one time, neurologists despaired of ever being able to limit stroke-related tissue destruction," say Drs. Justin Zivin and Dennis Choi, who have conducted pioneering research on tPA and the glutamate cascade. "Researchers have much to learn, but now there is reason for optimism."

Will African-Americans share such an optimistic future? The answer seems to be a qualified "yes." The National Institute of Neurological Disorders and Stroke is sponsoring several projects aimed specifically at the African-American community. At the University of Maryland at Baltimore, Dr. Steven Kittner is working to discover why the risk of stroke is so much higher for blacks, especially young adults (under age forty-five), than for whites. At Columbia University in New York City, Dr. Ralph Sacco is studying what causes strokes to recur in black and Hispanic patients. And at the University of Tennessee at Memphis, Dr. Kenneth Gaines is researching how differences in hypertension, diet, smoking habits, and socioeconomic status explain racial differences in blood chemistry, heart problems, and other stroke-related factors. Working with a team of investigators from six Southern medical schools, Dr. Gaines hopes to assemble the African-American equivalent of the Framingham study, whose participants were virtually all white. These and other research efforts will eventually help doctors understand how to tailor stroke prevention and treatment to the special needs of African-Americans.

On the other hand, many barriers that prevent black Americans from receiving optimal health care are stubborn indeed. In fact, the health care gap between the haves and have-nots may widen, according to Dr. Charles K. Francis of the Harlem Hospital Medical Center. "Political leaders support getting basic medical care to the inner cities, which is important. But you can't evaluate a stroke patient without CT or MRI technology, which is expensive—too expensive, many politicians say." Dr. Francis and others worry that in an era of rising health care costs, good health care is becoming increasingly available only to those who can afford it.

## THE PERSONAL ASSAULT ON STROKE

Fortunately, some of our best weapons against stroke don't depend on what technology or research labs can do for us. It's all about what we can do for ourselves. Most of the findings emerging from the nation's research labs deal with preventing the deadly or disabling aftermath of a stroke. But safeguarding our own health can help prevent strokes—and a host of other disabling diseases and conditions—from ever developing. Taking charge of our health helps us feel, look, and *be* better, stronger, more in control, more alive, and ultimately, happier.

While African-Americans are often underserved by the health care system, Dr. Louis Sullivan says the truly underserved are those of us who don't take care of ourselves. And that doesn't just mean physically, but mentally and spiritually, too. Addressing a class of medical school graduates, Secretary Sullivan offered this poignant reminder of our responsibility to ourselves:

> The availability of adequate health care is certainly a concern of government. Indeed, for many of the poor and elderly, it is the direct responsibility of the government. But no amount of health care is going to save peo-

ple from sickness or death if they drink too much, smoke, take drugs, don't exercise, don't eat a proper diet, and, most of all, don't seek regular medical care. We want to do everything we can to serve all Americans. But once they are served, we need to say to them, in effect: "Now it's your turn."

If you picked up this book because you were curious about stroke and wanted to learn more, we hope we have quenched your thirst. If you or someone you love has suffered a stroke, we hope these pages have helped you understand recovery and rehabilitation, and helped replace despair with a measure of hope. If you are at risk of a stroke and want to avoid one, or you simply want to lead a healthful, fuller lifestyle, we hope the book has given you powerful tools to forge a bountiful new way of living.

For generations, through tragedy and triumph, black people have managed to do what we've had to do to survive. Now we're turning a new page. Because today, survival means more than staying alive. It means being healthy.

Secretary Sullivan couldn't have advised us better. Now it's our turn.

# Myths About Stroke

| Myth | Fact |
|---|---|
| "A stroke can happen to anyone. Only fate determines who is hit." | A stroke is the end result of a long-term process. Uncontrolled hypertension, one of the leading causes of stroke in blacks, is usually present for many years before it bursts a blood vessel in the brain. The same is true for thickening and hardening of the arteries, also a cause of stroke. By attending to these underlying causes, strokes can be prevented. |

| Myth | Fact |
|------|------|
| "Tension is what causes high blood pressure. As long as you feel okay and you're not tense, you'll never have to worry about having a stroke." | Stress contributes to hypertension, but so do too much sodium and alcohol, too little exercise, being overweight, and other factors. Whether you have hypertension has nothing to do with how you feel, because hypertension doesn't have symptoms. So you can have high blood pressure whether you're tense or relaxed. |
| "Never bend down after a stroke. It will bring on another one." | A brain hemorrhage is caused by long-term untreated hypertension or a sudden significant increase in blood pressure. Bending down can cause a slight elevation in blood pressure inside the head, but if the patient is controlling blood pressure through diet, exercise, and medication, the risk of stroke is negligible. |
| "The third stroke always kills." | Some patients die after one stroke. Others live through several or more and return to normal life. |

| Myth | Fact |
|------|------|
| "Stroke patients should take it easy." | Patients should be encouraged to lead active, independent lives. It gives them an incentive to overcome their disability and contributes to a fuller recovery. |
| "Black people don't get heart disease." | Heart disease, a risk factor for stroke, now occurs nearly as often in black men as it does in white men. Black women actually have more heart disease than do white women. |

# Resources

## FOR GENERAL INFORMATION

Facts about stroke are easy to get. Pamphlets and other written materials are available for the asking; phone calls, many toll-free, can connect you with organizations that can answer general questions or refer you to someone who can.

**The National Stroke Association** is the only national health organization exclusively devoted to stroke prevention, treatment, and rehabilitation. NSA provides books, audio and videotapes, training programs, free or low-cost brochures, and other educational materials for patients, families, persons at risk, and medical professionals. NSA members receive a one-year subscription to *Be Smart* and a 10 percent discount on NSA materials. Membership also includes STROKE PREVENT, your personal stroke risk profile and prevention plan, as well as information on specialized products designed for stroke patients. Annual membership is $20, though NSA will enroll persons on fixed incomes regardless of donation level.

National Stroke Association
96 Inverness Drive, Suite I
Englewood, CO 80112
(800) STROKES [(800) 787-6537]
www.stroke.org

**The American Heart Association** has information for stroke patients and their families and friends on after-stroke care. AHA also has free brochures and pamphlets on aspects of stroke, such as *Stroke: A Guide for the Family* (a 25-page booklet that explains what a stroke is, treatment, recovery, and rehabilitation, with emphasis on how family members can help a patient recover). You can also get a free newsletter, *Stroke Connection*, published six times a year. Phone the AHA's Stroke Connection at (800) 553-6321 or look for their website at www.americanheart.org

## ALCOHOL

**Alcoholics Anonymous,** the oldest and most famous self-help group for persons struggling to control their drinking, is still among the most effective approaches. AA uses a 12-step program to help people recognize the nature of their relationship with alcohol, accept spiritual help as a guiding force, and make amends to the persons they have harmed. Alateen is for teens with drinking problems. Local Al-Anon and Alateen groups are found throughout the United States.

Alcoholics Anonymous World Services
475 Riverside Drive
New York, NY 10163
(212) 870-3400

Alateen
1600 Corporate Landing Parkway
Virginia Beach, VA 23454-5617
(757) 563-1600

## APHASIA

The nonprofit **National Aphasia Association** offers many publications, including "Aphasia Quiz" and "How to Communicate with a Person Who Has Aphasia." NAA also has a host of local support groups for aphasia patients; many are affiliated with stroke support groups, though the association points out that not every support group for stroke patients accepts persons with aphasia. Publications are free with a donation and stamps.

National Aphasia Association
156 Fifth Avenue, Suite 707
New York, NY 10010
(800) 922-4622 or (212) 255-4329
www.aphasia.org

To locate a qualified speech therapist near you, contact:

American Speech, Language, and Hearing Association
10801 Rockville Pike
Rockville, MD 20852
(800) 638-8255 or (301) 897-5700
www.asha.org

## DIABETES

The **National Diabetes Information Clearinghouse**, a service of the National Institutes of Health, can send you free educational materials, including nutrition information, a diabetes dictionary, a fact sheet on diabetes in African-Americans, and a directory of local diabetes-related programs for black Americans.

National Diabetes Information Clearinghouse
Box NDIC
Bethesda, MD 20892
(301) 654-3327
www.niddk.nih.org

## FREE OR LOW-COST MEDICINE

Many pharmaceutical companies have programs to help low-income patients obtain medicines free of charge or at low cost. Companies generally provide this service to patients who are not eligible for private or public health insurance, but there are exceptions. Usually your doctor contacts the company on your behalf. Information on patient-assistance programs for some of the most popular stroke-related medicines is given below. If you have access to the Internet, you'll find additional details at the following website: www.phrma.org/patients/index.html

### Blood Pressure Medicine

For information on antihypertension medicine made by **Lederle Laboratories**, ask your doctor to phone the Indigent Patient Program at (800) 568-9938.

**Boehringer Ingelheim Pharmaceuticals,** makers of Catapres and other blood pressure medicines, will send your doctor information on how to enroll you in their Partners in Health Program to obtain low-cost medication. In general, the program is open to patients who are not eligible for Medicaid or similar assistance programs and who meet the company's income eligibility rules. For information, call (800) 556-8317.

**Squibb Company,** makers of over a dozen heart medicines, offers free and low-cost medicine to qualified patients. For more information, call Squibb Customer Service at (800) 332-2056.

**Hoechst Marion Roussel,** makers of Cardizem, targets patients who have incomes below the federal poverty line and who are not eligible for a prescription reimbursement plan, including Medicaid. The company will mail an Indigent Patient Assistance Form to your doctor, who determines whether you are eligible for the program. For details, phone (800) 221-4025.

**Knoll Pharmaceuticals,** makers of Isoptin, will send you a three-month supply of medication at no charge. You can reapply for additional medicine at the end of three months. For application materials, ask your doctor to phone the company at (800) 524-2474.

**Merck & Co.,** makers of Diupres and Diuril, will send you a three-month supply of medicine through your doctor's office if you have no access to health insurance and you cannot afford prescription medicine.

Have your doctor phone (800) 994-2111 for an application form.

**Novartis,** makers of Apresolin, Esidrix, and other blood pressure medicines, makes certain medications available at reduced cost for qualified patients. Call (800) 257-3273 for details. The operator will ask you for your Social Security number, date of birth, address and phone number, medication and dosage, insurance information, monthly income and source, number of people in your home, and your doctor's name and address.

**Zeneca Pharmaceuticals,** makers of Sular, Tenoretic, Tenormin, and Zestril, will send you, your doctor, or a social worker application materials for its Patient Assistance Program. If you are accepted into the program, the company will deliver medicine to your home every three months for one year. You can reapply to the program after one year. The medicine is free; there is a $5 delivery charge. Call (302) 886-2231.

### Kidney Medicine

If you are on dialysis and you meet certain income and insurance requirements, **Amgen, Inc.**, will provide its kidney medicine, Epogen, at no charge to you. You will receive a twelve-month supply, after which your physician can reapply for an additional amount. Your doctor can enroll you in the Safety Net Program for Epogen by phone at (800) 272-9376.

## HYPERTENSION

You can get general information about high blood pressure by contacting:

National Heart, Lung, and Blood Institute
Building 31, Room 4A-21
Bethesda, MD 20892
(301) 496-4236
www.nhlbi.nih.gov

## REHABILITATION

Stroke clubs and stroke support groups help support patients through recovery and rehabilitation, and help family members cope with the new demands of caring for a stroke patient. Your local American Heart Association office can supply information on stroke clubs in your area, or advice on how to start one. The National Stroke Association also keeps a national listing of stroke clubs, and is interested in identifying support groups for young stroke patients. (For contact information, see the NSA listing under "For General information.") Hospitals that treat sizable numbers of stroke patients sometimes organize stroke support groups, too.

## RELAXATION THERAPY

You can learn relaxation therapy at any of hundreds of neighborhood health centers, schools, YMCAs and YWCAs, and hospitals and university medical centers across the country. You don't have to learn relaxation in a classroom, of course, but a group setting can be helpful for people who have difficulty relaxing or who find it difficult to get motivated without peer support.

## SMOKING

The **American Lung Association** has a program to encourage African-American smokers to quit. For more information, contact your local ALA office by dialing (800) LUNG-USA, or (800) 586-4872.

The **American Cancer Society** has information on smoking and cancer for African-Americans. Contact your local ACS office by dialing (800) ACS-2345, or (800) 227-2345.

The **National Cancer Institute** offers free publications and brief recorded messages about cancer. Phone (800) 4-CANCER, or (800) 422-6237. For more information, visit NCI's website at www.nci.nih.gov

# APPENDIX C

# Nutritive Value
# of Common Foods[†]

| | Amt | Calories | Protein (g) | Fat (g) | Carbohydrate (g) | Calcium (mg) | Phosphorus (mg) |
|---|---|---|---|---|---|---|---|
| **Milk** | | | | | | | |
| Buttermilk | 1 C | 88 | 8.8 | 0.2 | 12.5 | 296 | 233 |
| Milk, skim | 1 C | 88 | 8.8 | 0.2 | 12.5 | 296 | 233 |
| Milk, whole | 1 C | 159 | 8.5 | 8.5 | 12.0 | 288 | 227 |
| **Vegetables** | | | | | | | |
| *Asparagus | 4 | | | | | | |
| Green beans, frozen, french style | ½ C | 14 | 1.2 | 0.1 | 3.1 | 19 | 25 |
| Beans, lima (frozen) | ½ C | 84 | 5.1 | 0.1 | 16.2 | 17 | 77 |
| Beets | ½ C | 27 | 1.0 | 0.1 | 6.1 | 12 | 20 |
| *Beet greens, spinach, collards (cooked) | ½ C | 22 | 2.5 | 0.4 | 3.5 | 111 | 34 |
| *Brussels Sprouts, frozen | ½ C | | | | | | |
| Cabbage, raw | 1 C | 21 | 1.7 | 0.2 | 4.2 | 25 | 34 |
| Cauliflower | ½ C | | | | | | |
| Corn on cob, 5" (boiled) | 1 | 70 | 2.5 | 0.8 | 16.2 | 2 | 69 |
| Peas, green, frozen | ½ C | 55 | 4.1 | 0.3 | 9.5 | 15 | 69 |
| Potato, french fried (2" to 3 ½" diameter) | 10 | 137 | 2.2 | 6.6 | 18.0 | 8 | 56 |
| Potato, sweet, mashed | ¼ C | 73 | 1.1 | 0.3 | 16.8 | 21 | 30 |
| Potato, white, baked (2" diameter) | ½ C | 59 | 1.7 | 0.1 | 13.3 | 6 | 41 |
| *Pumpkin, carrots, winter squash | ½ C | 37 | 1.1 | 0.3 | 8.9 | 27 | 32 |
| Rutabagas, mashed | ½ C | 42 | 1.1 | 0.1 | 9.9 | 71 | 37 |
| *Summer squash | ½ C | | | | | | |

| Iron (mg) | Sodium (mg) | Potassium (mg) | Vit. A (IU) | Thiamine (mg) | Riboflavin (mg) | Niacin (mg) | Ascorbic Acid (mg) | USDA Handbook No.456 Ref. No. |
|---|---|---|---|---|---|---|---|---|
| 0.1 | 319 | 343 | 10 | 0.10 | 0.44 | 0.2 | 2 | 509b |
| 0.1 | 127 | 355 | 10 | 0.09 | 0.44 | 0.2 | 2 | 1322b |
| 0.1 | 122 | 351 | 350 | 0.07 | 0.41 | 0.2 | 2 | 1320b |
|  |  |  |  |  |  |  |  | 47b |
| 0.5 | 1 | 99 | 443 | 0.07 | 0.08 | 0.5 | 10 | 194c |
| 1.5 | 86 | 362 | 195 | 0.06 | 0.03 | 0.9 | 15 | 173c |
| 0.5 | 37 | 177 | 15 | 0.03 | 0.04 | 0.3 | 5 | 385b |
| 1.4 | 33 | 260 | 6133 | 0.07 | 0.14 | 0.6 | 36 | 393a, 2170a, 807a |
|  |  |  |  |  |  |  |  | 492c |
| 0.5 | 12 | 189 | 200 | 0.06 | 0.06 | 0.4 | 47 | 512c 631a |
| 0.5 | — | 151 | 310 | 0.09 | 0.08 | 1.1 | 7 | 846a |
| 1.5 | 92 | 108 | 480 | 0.22 | 0.07 | 1.4 | 11 | 1530c |
| 0.7 | 3 | 427 | — | 0.07 | 0.04 | 1.6 | 11 | 1789b |
| 0.5 | 7 | 155 | 5038 | 0.06 | 0.04 | 0.4 | 11 | 2250c |
| 0.5 | 3 | 316 | — | 0.07 | 0.03 | 1.2 | 13 | 1787d |
| 0.5 | 10 | 261 | 6757 | 0.04 | 0.08 | 0.6 | 7 | 1832d, 620a, 2201a |
| 0.4 | 5 | 201 | 660 | 0.07 | 0.07 | 1.0 | 31 | 1920b |
|  |  |  |  |  |  |  |  | 2192a |

| | Amt | Calo-ries | Pro-tein (g) | Fat (g) | Carbo-hydrate (g) | Cal-cium (mg) | Phos-phorus (mg) |
|---|---|---|---|---|---|---|---|
| Celery, stalks | 3 | | | | | | |
| Cucumber, slices | 16 | 9 | 0.7 | 0.1 | 2.1 | 19 | 17 |
| Lettuce, shredded | 1 C | | | | | | |
| *Tomatoes, canned and juice | ½ C | 24 | 1.2 | 0.2 | 5.2 | 8 | 23 |
| Tomatoes, fresh,(2 ²/₅" diameter) | 1 | 20 | 1.0 | 0.2 | 4.3 | 12 | 25 |
| Turnips, mashed | ½ C | 26 | 0.9 | 0.3 | 5.7 | 41 | 28 |
| **Fruits** | | | | | | | |
| Apple (2 ½" diameter) | 1 | 61 | 0.2 | 0.6 | 15.3 | 7 | 11 |
| Applesauce, unsweetened | ½ C | 50 | 0.3 | 0.3 | 13.2 | 5 | 6 |
| Banana, medium | ½ | 51 | 0.7 | 0.1 | 13.2 | 5 | 16 |
| *Berries (blue, black, raspberries) | ½ C | 46 | 0.8 | 0.4 | 10.9 | 19 | 15 |
| Cantaloupe (¼ of 6" diameter) | 1 C | 48 | 1.1 | 0.2 | 12.0 | 22 | 26 |
| Citrus Fruit: | | | | | | | |
| *Orange/ grapefruit juice | ½ C | | | | | | |
| Orange, small | 1 | 49 | 0.8 | 0.1 | 11.8 | 19 | 19 |
| Grapefruit | ½ | | | | | | |
| Cherries, large | 10 | 47 | 0.9 | 0.2 | 11.7 | 15 | 13 |
| Grapes | 12 | 41 | 0.4 | 0.2 | 10.4 | 7 | 12 |
| Pears, water pack | 1 | 50 | 0.4 | 0.4 | 12.8 | 8 | 10 |
| Raisins (1 ½ T) | ½ oz | 40 | 0.4 | — | 10.8 | 9 | 14 |
| Strawberries | 1 C | 55 | 1.0 | 0.7 | 12.5 | 31 | 31 |
| Watermelon, diced | 1 C | 42 | 0.8 | 0.3 | 10.2 | 11 | 16 |

| Iron (mg) | Sodium (mg) | Potassium (mg) | Vit. A (IU) | Thiamine (mg) | Riboflavin (mg) | Niacin (mg) | Ascorbic Acid (mg) | USDA Handbook No.456 Ref. No. |
|---|---|---|---|---|---|---|---|---|
| 0.6 | 18 | 133 | 290 | 0.03 | 0.04 | 0.3 | 6 | 637c 942d |
| 0.9 | 200 | 269 | 1028 | 0.06 | 0.04 | 0.9 | 20 | 1256c 2284d, 2288d |
| 0.5 | 3 | 222 | 820 | 0.05 | 0.04 | 0.6 | 21 | 2282c |
| 0.5 | 39 | 216 | — | 0.05 | 0.06 | 0.4 | 26 | 2353b |
| 0.3 | 1 | 116 | 100 | 0.03 | 0.02 | 0.1 | 4 | 13d |
| 0.6 | 3 | 95 | 50 | 0.03 | 0.01 | 0.1 | 1 | 28e |
| 0.4 | 1 | 220 | 115 | 0.03 | 0.04 | 0.4 | 6 | 141b |
| 0.8 | 1 | 113 | 118 | 0.02 | 0.04 | 0.4 | 10 | 424b, 418a, 1851a |
| 0.6 | 19 | 402 | 5440 | 0.06 | 0.05 | 1.0 | 53 | 1358c |
| 0.3 | 1 | 189 | 158 | 0.08 | 0.3 | 0.3 | 49 | 1421c 1053b 1437b, 1061a |
| 0.3 | 1 | 129 | 70 | 0.03 | 0.04 | 0.3 | 7 | 663b |
| 0.2 | 2 | 104 | 60 | 0.04 | 0.02 | 0.2 | 2 | 1085a |
| 0.4 | 2 | 136 | — | 0.02 | 0.04 | 0.2 | 2 | 1504e |
| 0.5 | 4 | 107 | — | 0.02 | 0.01 | 0.1 | — | 1846c |
| 1.5 | 1 | 244 | 90 | 0.04 | 0.10 | 0.9 | 88 | 2217e |
| 0.8 | 2 | 160 | 940 | 0.05 | 0.05 | 0.3 | 11 | 2424c |

| | Amt | Calories | Protein (g) | Fat (g) | Carbohydrate (g) | Calcium (mg) | Phosphorus (mg) |
|---|---|---|---|---|---|---|---|
| **Breads and Crackers,** Enriched | | | | | | | |
| Biscuit (2" diameter, 1 ¼" high) | 1 | 103 | 2.1 | 4.8 | 12.8 | 34 | 49 |
| Cornbread, piece (2 ½" x 2 ½" x 1 ⅜") | 1 | 178 | 3.8 | 5.8 | 27.5 | 133 | 209 |
| Frankfurter roll (6") | 1 | 119 | 3.3 | 2.2 | 21.2 | 30 | 34 |
| Graham crackers | 2 | 55 | 1.1 | 1.3 | 10.4 | 6 | 21 |
| Hamburger bun (3 ½") | 1 | 119 | 3.3 | 2.2 | 21.2 | 30 | 34 |
| Muffin, plain (2" x 1 ½") | 1 | 118 | 3.1 | 4.0 | 16.9 | 42 | 60 |
| Saltines (2 ½" x square) | 4 | 48 | 1.0 | 1.3 | 8.0 | 2 | 10 |
| Soda crackers (2 ½" square) | 5 | 65 | 1.3 | 1.8 | 10.0 | 3 | 13 |
| White or whole wheat bread, slice | 1 | 76 | 2.4 | 0.9 | 14.1 | 24 | 27 |
| Bran flakes, 40% | ½ C | | | | | | |
| Corn flakes | ¾ C | 73 | 1.5 | 0.1 | 15.9 | — | 7 |
| Farina, cooked | ½ C | 51 | 1.6 | 0.1 | 10.6 | 5 | 15 |
| Grits, corn | ½ C | 62 | 1.4 | 0.1 | 13.5 | 1 | 13 |
| Oatmeal, cooked | ½ C | 66 | 2.4 | 1.2 | 11.6 | 11 | 68 |
| Rice, cooked | ⅓ C | 74 | 1.4 | 0.1 | 16.4 | 7 | 19 |
| Wheat, puffed | 1 C | 54 | 2.3 | 0.2 | 11.8 | 4 | 48 |
| **Pasta,** Enriched | | | | | | | |
| *Noodles, macaroni, spaghetti | ½ C | 91 | 3.0 | 0.6 | 18.3 | 7 | 41 |
| **Meat, Poultry, Fish** | | | | | | | |
| *Beef, lamb, veal | 1 oz | 79 | 7.4 | 5.2 | — | 3 | 32 |

| Iron (mg) | Sodium (mg) | Potassium (mg) | Vit. A (IU) | Thiamine (mg) | Riboflavin (mg) | Niacin (mg) | Ascorbic Acid (mg) | USDA Handbook No.456 Ref. No. |
|---|---|---|---|---|---|---|---|---|
| 0.4 | 175 | 33 | — | 0.06 | 0.06 | 0.5 | — | 410a |
| 0.8 | 263 | 61 | 130 | 0.10 | 0.10 | 0.8 | — | 1350d |
| 0.8 | 202 | 38 | — | 0.11 | 0.07 | 0.9 | — | 1902c |
| 0.2 | 95 | 55 | — | 0.01 | 0.03 | 0.2 | — | 914b |
| 0.8 | 202 | 38 | — | 0.11 | 0.07 | 0.9 | — | 1902c |
| 0.6 | 176 | 50 | 40 | 0.07 | 0.09 | 0.6 | — | 1343b |
| 0.1 | 123 | 13 | — | — | — | 0.1 | — | 916d |
| 0.2 | 156 | 16 | — | — | — | 0.1 | — | 918d |
| 0.7 | 142 | 29 | — | 0.07 | 0.06 | 0.7 | — | 461b |
| 0.4 | 188 | 22 | 885 | 0.22 | 0.26 | 2.2 | 7 | 866a |
| — | 176 | 11 | — | 0.05 | 0.03 | 0.5 | — | 992 |
| 0.4 | 251 | 14 | 75 | 0.05 | 0.04 | 0.5 | — | 863a |
| 0.7 | 262 | 73 | — | 0.09 | 0.02 | 0.1 | — | 1391 |
| 0.6 | 256 | 19 | — | 0.08 | 0.01 | 0.7 | — | 1872a |
| 0.6 | 1 | 51 | — | 0.08 | 0.03 | 1.2 | — | 2458 |
| 0.7 | 1 | 43 | — | 0.11 | 0.07 | 1.2 | — | 1378c, 1299c, 2159c |
| 0.8 | 16 | 74 | 2 | 0.03 | 0.07 | 1.6 | — | 353d, 1185e, 2370e |

| | Amt | Calo-ries | Pro-tein (g) | Fat (g) | Carbo-hydrate (g) | Cal-cium (mg) | Phos-phorus (mg) |
|---|---|---|---|---|---|---|---|
| Beef liver | 1 oz | 65 | 7.5 | 3.0 | 1.5 | 3 | 135 |
| Bologna (1 slice, 4 ½" diameter) | 1 oz | 86 | 3.4 | 7.8 | 0.3 | 2 | 36 |
| Chicken, light meat | 1 oz | 50 | 9.4 | 1.0 | — | 3 | 80 |
| *Cod, haddock, halibut (broiled) | 1 oz | 48 | 6.9 | 1.8 | 0.5 | 8 | 73 |
| Ham, cured | 1 oz | 92 | 6.3 | 7.1 | — | 3 | 52 |
| Hot dog | 1 | 139 | 5.6 | 12.4 | 0.8 | 3 | 60 |
| Pork, fresh | 1 oz | 103 | 6.8 | 8.1 | — | 3 | 73 |
| Shrimp | 1 oz | 37 | 7.7 | 0.4 | 0.2 | 37 | 84 |
| Tuna, canned in oil | 1 oz | 82 | 6.9 | 5.8 | — | 2 | 83 |
| **Egg,** large | 1 | 82 | 6.5 | 5.8 | 0.5 | 27 | 103 |
| **Cheese** | | | | | | | |
| Cheddar, domestic | 1 oz | 113 | 7.1 | 9.1 | 0.6 | 213 | 136 |
| Cottage cheese, small curd, creamed | ½ C | 112 | 14.3 | 4.4 | 3.1 | 98 | 160 |
| **Peanut Butter** | 2 T | 188 | 8.0 | 16.2 | 6.0 | 18 | 122 |
| **Dried Beans and Peas** | | | | | | | |
| *Navy beans, kidney beans, split peas | ½ C | 114 | 7.5 | 0.4 | 20.6 | 32 | 123 |
| **Fats** | | | | | | | |
| Bacon, crisp, slices | 2 | 86 | 3.8 | 7.8 | 0.5 | 2 | 34 |
| *Cream, light, 20% or half & half | 1 T | 26 | 0.5 | 2.5 | 0.7 | 16 | 13 |
| *French or Italian dressing | 1 T | 75 | 0.1 | 7.6 | 1.9 | 2 | 2 |
| *Margarine/butter | 1 t | 34 | — | 3.8 | — | 1 | 1 |

| Iron (mg) | Sodium (mg) | Potassium (mg) | Vit. A (IU) | Thiamine (mg) | Riboflavin (mg) | Niacin (mg) | Ascorbic Acid (mg) | USDA Handbook No.456 Ref. No. |
|---|---|---|---|---|---|---|---|---|
| 2.5 | 52 | 108 | 15130 | 0.07 | 1.19 | 4.7 | 7.7 | 1267a |
| 0.5 | 369 | 65 | — | 0.05 | 0.06 | 0.7 | — | 1982g |
| 0.4 | 19 | 123 | 17 | 0.01 | 0.02 | 3.5 | — | 682d |
| 0.3 | 40 | 121 | 80 | 0.01 | 0.02 | 1.4 | — | 795d, 1110d, 1104d |
| 0.8 | 227 | 71 | — | 0.15 | 0.06 | 1.1 | — | 1779f |
| 0.9 | 495 | 99 | — | 0.07 | 0.09 | 1.2 | — | 1994c |
| 0.9 | 17 | 78 | — | 0.26 | 0.07 | 1.6 | — | 1716e |
| 1.0 | — | 39 | 20 | — | 0.01 | 0.6 | — | 2045c |
| 0.3 | 227 | 85 | 26 | 0.01 | 0.02 | 2.9 | — | 2323h |
| 1.2 | 61 | 65 | 590 | 0.05 | 0.15 | — | — | 968b |
| 0.3 | 198 | 23 | 370 | 0.01 | 0.13 | — | — | 646p |
| 0.3 | 241 | 90 | 180 | 0.03 | 0.26 | 0.1 | — | 647d |
| 0.6 | 194 | 200 | — | 0.04 | 0.04 | 4.8 | — | 1499f |
| 2.2 | 8 | 342 | 15 | 0.12 | 0.07 | 0.8 | — | 115b, 161d, 1533a |
| 0.5 | 153 | 35 | — | 0.08 | 0.05 | 0.8 | — | 126d |
| — | 7 | 19 | 100 | — | 0.02 | — | — | 929b, 928b |
| 0.1 | 267 | 8 | — | — | — | — | — | 1932b, 1936b |
| — | 46 | 1 | 160 | — | — | — | — | 1317d, 505d |

|  | Amt | Calo-ries | Pro-tein (g) | Fat (g) | Carbo-hydrate (g) | Cal-cium (mg) | Phos-phorus (mg) |
|---|---|---|---|---|---|---|---|
| *Mayonnaise, salad dressing | 1 T | 83 | 0.2 | 8.8 | 1.3 | 3 | 4 |
| Oils | 1 T | 120 | — | 13.6 | — | — | — |
| **Nuts** | | | | | | | |
| *Unsalted peanuts, pecans, walnuts, almonds | 2 T | 103 | 2.9 | 9.6 | 2.9 | 20 | 64 |
| **Desserts** | | | | | | | |
| Brownies, with nuts (1 1/4" x 1 3/4" x 7/8") | 1 | 97 | 1.3 | 6.3 | 10.2 | 8 | 30 |
| Cake, chocolate (3" x 3" x 2") | 1 piece | 322 | 4.2 | 15.1 | 45.8 | 65 | 121 |
| Cake, plain (3" x 3" x 2") | 1 piece | 313 | 3.9 | 12.0 | 48.1 | 55 | 88 |
| Chocolate pudding | 1/2 C | 193 | 4.1 | 6.1 | 33.4 | 125 | 128 |
| Cookies, chocolate chip | 2 | 99 | 1.1 | 4.4 | 14.6 | 8 | 24 |
| Custard, baked | 1/2 C | 153 | 7.2 | 7.3 | 14.7 | 149 | 155 |
| Gelatin dessert | 1/2 C | 71 | 1.8 | — | 16.9 | — | — |
| Ice cream, vanilla | 4 fl oz | 129 | 3.0 | 7.0 | 13.9 | 97 | 77 |
| Pie, apple (9z diameter) | 1/8 pie | 302 | 2.6 | 13.1 | 45.0 | 9 | 26 |
| Sherbet, orange | 4 fl oz | 130 | 0.9 | 1.2 | 29.7 | 16 | 13 |
| Vanilla wafers | 5 | 93 | 1.1 | 3.2 | 14.9 | 8 | 13 |

| Iron (mg) | Sodium (mg) | Potassium (mg) | Vit. A (IU) | Thiamine (mg) | Riboflavin (mg) | Niacin (mg) | Ascorbic Acid (mg) | USDA Handbook No.456 Ref. No. |
|---|---|---|---|---|---|---|---|---|
| 0.1 | 86 | 3 | 35 | — | — | — | — | 1938b, 1940b |
| — | — | — | — | — | — | — | — | 1401j |
| 0.5 | 19 | 102 | 5 | 0.07 | 0.05 | 1.0 | — | 1496b, 1536j, 2421e, 8f |
| 0.4 | 50 | 38 | 40 | 0.04 | 0.02 | 0.1 | — | 813 |
| 0.8 | 259 | 123 | 130 | 0.02 | 0.09 | 0.2 | — | 525c |
| 0.3 | 258 | 68 | 150 | 0.02 | 0.08 | 0.2 | — | 534b |
| 0.7 | 73 | 223 | 195 | 0.03 | 0.18 | 0.2 | — | 1823 |
| 0.4 | 84 | 28 | 26 | 0.01 | 0.01 | 0.1 | — | 818b |
| 0.6 | 105 | 194 | 465 | 0.06 | 0.25 | 0.2 | — | 948 |
| — | 61 | — | — | — | — | — | — | 1032b |
| 0.1 | 42 | 121 | 295 | 0.03 | 0.14 | 0.1 | — | 1139d |
| 0.4 | 355 | 94 | 40 | 0.02 | 0.02 | 0.5 | 1 | 1566c |
| — | 10 | 21 | 60 | 0.01 | 0.03 | — | 2 | 2041b |
| 0.1 | 51 | 15 | 25 | 0.01 | 0.02 | 0.1 | — | 833b |

| | Amt | Calories | Protein (g) | Fat (g) | Carbohydrate (g) | Calcium (mg) | Phosphorus (mg) |
|---|---|---|---|---|---|---|---|
| **Sweets** | | | | | | | |
| Milk chocolate | 1 oz | 147 | 2.2 | 9.2 | 16.1 | 65 | 65 |
| *Molasses, jams, jelly, maple syrup | 1 T | 52 | 0.1 | — | 13.4 | 16 | 3 |
| Soft drinks | 6 fl oz | 72 | — | — | 18.5 | — | — |
| Sugar | 1 T | 46 | — | — | 11.9 | — | — |

+Approximate values. All values have been rounded to the nearest decimal point.
*Average value for the group of foods listed.
—Contributes in serving size indicated only trace amount of nutrient.

| Iron (mg) | Sodium (mg) | Potassium (mg) | Vit. A (IU) | Thiamine (mg) | Riboflavin (mg) | Niacin (mg) | Ascorbic Acid (mg) | USDA Handbook No.456 Ref. No. |
|---|---|---|---|---|---|---|---|---|
| 0.3 | 27 | 109 | 80 | 0.02 | 0.10 | 0.1 | — | 587 |
| 0.8 | 2 | 17 | — | — | 0.01 | — | — | 2050b, 1148e, 1149e, 2049d |
| — | — | — | — | — | — | — | — | 404a |
| — | — | — | — | — | — | — | — | 2230b |

# Glossary

**ADL:** Activities of daily living (bathing, grooming, eating, using a toilet, etc.).

**Agnosia:** Inability to recognize.

**Aneurism:** A bulge caused by a weak spot in the wall of an artery.

**Anomia:** Inability to name.

**Aphasia:** Difficulty understanding spoken and written words and in finding words to express one's self.

**Apraxia:** Inability to perform learned movements.

**Arteriovenous (AV) malformation:** An inherited condition in which arteries and veins are joined directly to each other instead of being joined by capillaries.

**Asterixis:** Intermittent inability of the muscles to sustain a person's posture.

**Atherosclerosis:** Thickening and narrowing of arteries by fatty plaque.

**Atrial fibrillation:** A condition in which heart chambers quiver instead of pumping in unison.

**Beta blocker:** A class of sympathetic depressant medicines used to lower blood pressure.

**Bruit:** An abnormal sound heard through a stethoscope

when blood passes through a blood vessel that is narrowed by plaque.

**Calcium-channel blocker**: Medicine that reduces high blood pressure by relaxing the blood vessels. It works by preventing calcium (which is needed for muscle contraction) from entering muscles that surround the arteries.

**Catheter:** A slender flexible tube inserted into the urinary tract (or with a condom over a man's penis) to collect urine.

**Cerebral hemorrhage** (also called **intracerebral hemorrhage**): Bleeding into the brain.

**Cerebrovascular:** Relating to blood vessels in the head.

**Contracture:** An involuntary muscle spasm caused by a stroke.

**Coronary artery disease:** Thickening and narrowing of the arteries that serve the heart.

**Dementia:** Mental deterioration.

**Diastole:** Relaxation of the heart between beats.

**Diastolic:** Blood pressure when the heart relaxes. It is the lower of the two numbers that measure blood presure.

**Diuretic:** Medicine that lowers high blood pressure by decreasing the amount of fluid in the body.

**Embolism:** An ischemic stroke caused by a blood clot or plaque that lodges in the brain after forming elsewhere in the body.

**Endocarditis:** Inflammation of the membrane surrounding the heart.

**Endothelial cell:** The protective inner lining of a blood vessel.

**Fibrinogen:** Protein that helps blood clot.

**Frontal lobe:** The front of the brain. It governs our emotions.

**Glutamate cascade:** A chain reaction of chemical events triggered by a stroke. It eventually kills brain neurons.

**Glutamate-receptor blocker:** Medicine that prevents glutamate, a stimulant released from dying neurons during a stroke, from attaching to other neurons and killing them during the glutamate cascade.

**Hemiparesis:** Paralysis on one side of the body.

**Hemoglobin:** The iron-containing pigment that binds oxygen to red blood cells.

**Hemorrhage:** Bleeding.

**Hemorrhagic stroke:** Bleeding into the brain (cerebral hemorrhage) or into the membrane between the brain and the inside of the skull (subarachnoid hemorrhage).

**Hypertension:** High blood pressure.

**Hypertensive:** 1. Referring to high blood pressure. 2. A person with high blood pressure.

**Ischemia:** Too little blood in a part of the body, caused by blockage of blood flow.

**Ischemic stroke:** Blockage of blood flow to the brain by a blood clot or fatty deposit.

**Lacunar stroke:** Brain damage caused by lacunae.

**Lacune:** A small pit or cavity in brain tissue caused by the pressure of a small clot pressing outward from inside a blood vessel.

**Left ventricular hypertrophy:** Enlargement of the left side of the heart (the left ventricle).

**Mitral valve prolapse:** A heart condition in which the valves do not make a complete seal with surrounding tissue.

**Motor neurons:** Nerves responsible for sending messages to muscles and glands.

**Neuron:** A nerve cell.

**Normotensive:** 1. Normal blood pressure. 2. A person with normal blood pressure.

**Occipital lobe:** The back of the brain. It is responsible for vision.

**Plaque:** A yellowish fatty material that can build up inside blood vessels to the point of obstructing blood flow. Plaque is made of cholesterol, red blood cells, and bloodstream debris.

**Plasticity:** The ability of the brain to compensate for an injury.

**Platelet:** A red blood cell responsible for clotting.

**Pulmonary embolism:** The lodging of a blood clot in the artery that feeds blood to the lungs.

**Sensory neurons:** Nerves responsible for receiving information about light, heart, presure, and other stimuli.

**Stepped care:** An approach to managing high blood pressure by starting a patient with a diuretic and adding additional medicines until hypertension is controlled.

**Subarachnoid hemorrhage:** Bleeding into the membrane (the subarachnoid space) between the brain and the inside of the skull.

**Sympathetic depressant:** Medicine that reduces high blood pressure by helping the heart pump less blood and relaxing the blood vessels.

**Systole:** Contraction of the heart.

**Systolic:** The blood pressure reading when the heart contracts. It is the higher of the two numbers that measure blood pressure.

**Temporal lobe:** The middle portion of the brain. It controls smell, taste, hearing, memory, and certain visual associations.

**Thrombosis:** An ischemic stroke caused by a blood clot of plaque formed at the site of the blockage.

**TIA (Transient Ischemic Attack):** Brief blockage of a blood vessel in the brain by a clot or plaque that dissolves, usually within minutes, thereby restoring blood flow.

**Vasodilator:** Medicine that reduces high blood pressure by widening the blood vessels.

# Index

# About the Authors

LaFayette Singleton, M.D., is a neurologist at Cook County Hospital, Chicago, and a member of the American Association of Neurophysiology. Previously, he was an attending neurologist at Chicago's St. Mary of Nazareth Hospital and also served as a clinical assistant professor at Chicago Medical School.

Kirk A. Johnson is founding editor of the award-winning *Journal of Health Care for the Poor and Underserved,* published by Meharry Medical College in Nashville, Tenn. He was senior researcher on the PBS civil-rights documentary "Eyes on the Prize," and has testified before Congress on health protection for minorities. His work appears in national publications such as *Heart & Soul, Essence, HealthQuest,* and *Columbia Journalism Review.*

Linda Villarosa is an editor in the Science Department of the *New York Times* and former executive editor of *Essence* magazine. She is also the author of three books, including *Body & Soul: The Black Women's Guide to Physical Health and Emotional Well-Being.*

Maudene Nelson, M.S., R.D., a registered dietition and certified diabetes educator, is a staff associate at the Institute of Human Nutrition, College of Physicians & Surgeons, Columbia University, and a nutritionist for the Arteriosclerosis Research Center at Columbia-Presbyterian Medical Center.

# New Perspectives in Health Care from Kensington Books

# Parenting Advice

__Baby: An Owner's Manual__ $14.00US/$17.00CAN
By Bud Zukow, M.D. and Nancy Kaneshiro 1-57566-055-5
Dr. Zukow has been fielding parents' most common (and not-so-common) pediatric questions for more than 30 years. From ground zero through the end of the first year, this wise, witty, indispensible book provides answers and practical tips for your most pressing problems.

__How to Get the Best Public Education for Your Child__
*A Practical Parent's Guide for the 1990's* $4.50US/$5.50CAN
By Carol A. Ryan & Paula Sline with Barbara Lagowski 0-8217-4038-5
Here is an insider's perspective combining general information with specific advice. The book includes how to select the best school for your child, how to judge your child's progress, and how to evaluate their teachers. Written by two authors with over 40 years of combined experience in education, this guide will help children fulfill their potential.

__Stepparenting__
*Everything You Need to Know to Make it Work* $13.00US/$16.00CAN
By Jeanette Lofas, CSW, with Dawn B. Sova 1-57566-113-6
Practical, current advice for dealing with the many baffling issues that beset today's stepfamilies. From dating to remarriage, from stepsibling rivalry to joint custody, here is an invaluable resource for coping with today's most complex challenges. Discover the techniques, tools, and strategies that break through the barriers and lead to familial harmony.

---

Call toll free **1-888-345-BOOK** to order by phone or use this coupon to order by mail.

Name _____

Address _____

City _____ State _____ Zip _____

Please send me the books I have checked above.

I am enclosing $_____

Plus postage and handling* $_____

Sales tax (in New York and Tennessee) $_____

Total amount enclosed $_____

*Add $2.50 for the first book and $.50 for each additional book.

Send check or money order (no cash or CODs) to:

**Kensington Publishing Corp., 850 Third Avenue, New York, NY 10022**

Prices and Numbers subject to change without notice.

All orders subject to availability.

Check out our website at **www.kensingtonbooks.com**

# Mickey Rawlings Mysteries
# By Troy Soos

__**Hunting a Detroit Tiger**        $5.99US/$7.50CAN
    1-57566-291-4

__**Murder at Ebbets Field**        $4.99US/$5.99CAN
    1-57566-027-X

__**Murder at Fenway Park**        $4.99US/$5.99CAN
    0-8217-4909-9

__**Murder at Wrigley Field**        $5.50US/$7.00CAN
    1-57566-155-1

---

# THRILLS AND CHILLS
## The Mysteries of Mary Roberts Rinehart